CHICAGO PUBLIC LIBRARY
HAROLD WASHINGTON LIBRARY CENTER

R00164 88622

R00164 8862

W9-CFP-567

Blood droplets, indicating direction of fall

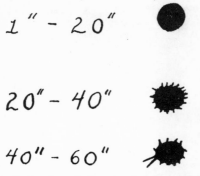

1″ - 20″

20″ - 40″

40″ - 60″

Blood droplets, indicating height of fall

OUTLINE OF DEATH INVESTIGATION

Outline of
Death Investigation

Second Printing

By

RAYMOND I. HARRIS, LL.B.

Coroner of St. Louis County
Formerly Assistant Attorney General
Former Magistrate Judge of St. Louis County
St. Louis, Missouri

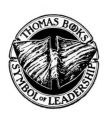

CHARLES C THOMAS • **PUBLISHER**

Springfield • *Illinois* • *U.S.A.*

REF
RA
1063
.H28
cop. 1

Published and Distributed Throughout the World by
CHARLES C THOMAS • PUBLISHER
Bannerstone House
301-327 East Lawrence Avenue, Springfield, Illinois, U.S.A.

This book is protected by copyright. No part of it
may be reproduced in any manner without written
permission from the publisher.

© *1962, by* CHARLES C THOMAS • PUBLISHER
ISBN 0-398-00784-5
Library of Congress Catalog Card Number: 62-16440

First Printing, 1962
Second Printing, 1973

*With THOMAS BOOKS careful attention is given to all details of
manufacturing and design. It is the Publisher's desire to present books that are
satisfactory as to their physical qualities and artistic possibilities and
appropriate for their particular use. THOMAS BOOKS will be true to those
laws of quality that assure a good name and good will.*

Printed in the United States of America
R-1

APR 2 1 1977

Dedicated to my wife, Lil, with thanks for her help, encouragement and patience during the time it has taken to assemble and prepare this manuscript.

PREFACE

When pilots get into their large aircraft, they use a check list as a guaranty against overlooking a step necessary in the operation of a plane. Their use of this safeguard does not indicate lack of knowledge on their part or lack of confidence in their abilities. Contrariwise, their thorough background, know-how and capabilities have proven that, as human beings, they are susceptible to error, and that memory refreshers and check list are important to protect against this human error during a technical operation where one oversight or one mistep could conceivably lead to disaster.

Investigation of deaths is analogous to the above situation. The expert investigator realizes that when he authorizes the removal of a body or permits its autopsy, embalming or cremation, or when he allows any possible evidence or clues to be disturbed or clothes from the corpse removed, he has taken a step on a path that cannot be retraced, and he has destroyed all possibilities of further investigation, examination or reconstruction of that phase of investigation; he further realizes that in permitting any of the above steps, he has contaminated, mutilated, liquidated and rendered helpless evidence or clues that might have been all-important in a final solution and desired prosecution.

Certainly, it then becomes logical and proper to use a check list or notebook to refresh the memory, outline the course of action, enumerate the essentials of any particular crime, and set forth the clues and evidence necessary to guide and aid the investigator. Finally, it must be realized, particularly in rural communities and smaller cities and counties, that an officer or coroner acting as an investigator may handle any one particular type of death very seldom, if only once in his career. Thusly, regardless of the amount of periodicals and textbooks that he has read or seminars and conventions that he has attended, it is impossible for him to retain all of the information, knowledge and know-how, especially in a technical line, as a matter of memory alone.

Taking these factors into consideration, this book has been prepared for coroners and investigators, not as a technical text book but rather as a ready reference to refresh their memory, outline their procedure, set forth particulars necessary in investigation and as a check list to be used at the scene, during the investigation and in preparation for submission of the case to other law authorities or for trial.

This book is divided into the following categories: pictures to be used for comparison and explanation, charts to be used for reference, forms to be used as guide and check list, and glossary to be used as a quick reference to definitions and a right hand to proper spelling in report preparation, outlines to be used on the scene and during the investigation itself, and short synopses for general information.

This author is well aware of the fact that death and homicide are almost as old as the world itself, and that the first murder case dates back thousands and thousands of years to the slewing of Abel by Cain. Certainly, in the multitude of years that have passed there have been many millions of investigations of all types of death and thousands of books and articles written about same. This work does not attempt to bring about any new miracle of investigation or any startling innovations in investigative procedure, but merely to accomplish the purposes set forth in the preceding paragraph.

With the cooperation of the publisher and with these purposes in mind, this work is prepared in a short, concise, simplified manner, and so published and bound as to make it convenient to be carried in the compartment of an emergency or squad car and on the person of an investigating official.

ACKNOWLEDGMENTS

This brief space and few words devoted to their recognition should not be taken as the measure of my appreciation of the encouragement, assistance and cooperation which I have received and without which I could not have written this book.

I wish particularly to acknowledge my thanks and appreciation to my secretary and administrative assistant, Mildred B. Saemann, for her invaluable assistance and her magnanimous contribution of time during her non-working hours in helping me assemble this text and in typing and editing its entire contents.

My sincere thanks also to Sheryn Goldenhersh for her art work; to Dr. Eugene Tucker, M.D., Pathologist, for material furnished and expert advice; to Dr. Edward Hunter, D.D.S., for his aid in connection with the section on teeth; to Richard Rose, Photographer; to the St. Louis Office of the Federal Bureau of Investigation and Missouri State Highway Patrol for supplying literature pertaining to collection, preservation and shipping of evidence; and, finally, to the many others who helped me collect material and illustrations necessary to complete this book.

R. I. H.

CONTENTS

OUTLINE OF DEATH INVESTIGATION

INTRODUCTION

The office of the coroner is an ancient one, having its birth in England many centuries ago. Originally, men of noble blood, who were close to and trusted by the King, were appointed to that position (originally called Corona) to investigate unexpected deaths and, as personal representatives and appointees of the King, to claim certain properties for the Crown.

The office of the coroner was transplanted to America by the English colonists, as were many of the English usages and laws.

In the three centuries that this office has existed in America it has undergone many changes in the various states to the present where there are almost as many different types of coroner's offices in the United States as there are states; a review of these various jurisdictions indicates that the coroner's system differs widely in qualifications of officials, their duties and selection.

The majority of states still retain the old coroner's laws with slight changes. Other states have either a medical examiner or a combination of both coroner and medical examiner. In most of the states the coroner is still elected for a two or four year term by the county in which he resides; in a few states he is appointed. In others the medical examiner is appointed locally, while in a few he is appointed by the Governor or by a chief state pathologist. It should be noted that the coroner's duties vary in the different jurisdictions from simple medical examination to a combination of medical examination and factual investigation to full law enforcement—from an office composed of one part time official to a multi-employee million dollar a year scientific-legal-investigative project. In some states the coroner has jurisdiction over the incompetent and insane, the raped and the molested; in others he also performs certain functions of the sheriff.

Which of the various offices is preferable is a question that still has not been answered by law enforcement, legal or medical authorities. It must be concluded that the operation and efficiency of the office depends upon the person himself, and that an efficient coroner's office or medical examiner's office requires both a medical and a legal knowledge in order: (1) to determine the cause of death, (2) to supervise proper investigation, and (3) effectuate law enforcement.

"If he is untrained, his mistaken verdicts can convict the innocent and set the murderers free." It is the duty of the coroner's office to properly examine and when necessary autopsy all subjects. X-ray examination and toxicological examinations are a must where the causes of death are not reasonably certain. Murder can easily be hidden and murderers can travel freely in society because a death has not been properly reviewed by efficient pathological, X-ray and toxicological experts or because of a lack of proper scientific and testing equipment to aid these experts. A factual report to these experts before the autopsy can help them determine what evidence is relevant and important. Medical examination must be accompanied by detailed investigation of the circumstances surrounding the death. The evidence available at the time of this investigation must be properly accumulated, digested and recorded so that none of it is misunderstood, mutilated, destroyed or improperly used, guaranteeing that when a crime exists it may be discovered and officials may conduct efficient prosecution at a later date.

It is also the duty of the coroner and his staff not merely to recognize crime and aid in convicting and punishing the guilty, but also to gather evidence necessary in establishing whether the death be accidental, suicidal, homicidal or natural. It is further their duty to completely explain and report the facts, so that the innocent may be protected, the reputation of families secured and the dead properly represented.

The coroner has a further duty of digesting the findings in any one or group of investigations, views or inquests, and utilizing them by transmitting the information gained therefrom to the proper authorities, for the purpose of eliminating any such deaths in the future.

Numerous accidents and deaths, because of dangerous conditions, can be minimized if the coroner, in addition to his other duties, considers himself a civic officer and pursues the reporting of the needed changes to the proper officials and to the public generally.

The coroner's office can best approach perfection where it maintains proper and complete cooperation and co-ordination with the medical units and police officials of the county, and the community generally. When these groups cooperate and coordinate their information and utilize their combined influence to effectuate efficiency, the community benefits, because unnecessary deaths and injuries are eliminated, because past deaths serve a purpose in the sense that such future deaths and resulting catastrophes may be averted, and, finally, because the innocent are protected and the guilty properly punished.

—1—

HOMICIDE LAW

I. General
- A. Definition
  Killing of one human being by another
- B. History
  1. Based on Common Law (unwritten law of England prior to establishment of States)
  2. Further explained and modified by Statutes, or State Laws

II. Kinds
- A. Felonious
  1. Murder
     a. Definition
        Killing of one human being by another with malice aforethought
        (1) Malice may or may not be accompanied by ill will
        (2) Malice may be expressed or implied
            (a) Implied malice
                Where act that is committed would have a tendency to kill somebody
            (b) Felony-Murder Doctrine
                The killing of somebody while engaging in the commission of a felony

6

Note: Important if that type of
felony is dangerous to others
AND
Whether the act committed
is the proximate cause of the
death

b. Degrees of murder
   (1) At Common Law there were no
   degrees of murder
   Note: Dividing line was deliberation and premeditation
c. Under Modern Laws usually 1st and
   2nd Degrees of murder

2. Manslaughter
   a. Culpable negligence
   b. Assisting another in the commission
   of self murder (suicide)
   c. Killing of an unborn quick child by
   injury to the mother, if such injury to
   the mother would be murder if her
   death resulted therefrom
   d. Abortion or intentional miscarriage
   resulting in death to the mother
   e. Death from a vicious animal
   f. Intoxicated physician administering
   drugs or medications, from which
   death results

Note: Classification of manslaughter
   a. Voluntary
      (1) Intentional
      (2) Without malice
      (3) Committed in heat of passion
      (4) When act is urged by adequate
      provocation

      b. Involuntary manslaughter
         (1) Unintentional
         (2) Without justification
         (3) Without excuse
         (4) Without malice

B. Non-felonious
  1. Justifiable homicide
    a. Definition
      Committed with intent but under circumstances of duty as to render the act proper
    b. Examples
      (1) Self defense
      (2) Defense of a relative, where he is without fault in provoking the conflict
      (3) Preventing the commission of a felony
      (4) Killing of a felon to prevent escape
     Note: Cannot kill to prevent escape of a person who has committed a misdemeanor
      (5) Suppressing a riot
      (6) Lawfully keeping or preserving the peace
      (7) Execution of a condemned person
  2. Excusable
    a. Definition
      Under circumstances of accident or necessity, where the party cannot strictly be said to have committed the act wilfully or intentionally

b. Examples
    (1) During the lawful and reasonable correcting of a child or servant
    (2) In the heat of passion
        (a) Upon sudden provocation
        AND
        (b) Without undue advantage being taken
        AND
        (c) Without a dangerous weapon
        AND
        (d) Not done in a cruel or unusual way or manner

C. Accidental
  1. Definition
    a. Happening by chance or unexpected
    AND
    b. Without foresight or expectation
    AND
    c. Without design or intent

—2—

INVESTIGATIVE PROCEDURE
SYNOPSIS

Common sense should guide the investigator in conducting his investigation, and some emergencies may call for various types of action; for example, where death may occur in a schoolyard or in a crowded area it is permissible to cover the body with a sheet or blanket which will keep same from the view of innocent bystanders and yet will not destroy any evidence, if carefully done. The chalking of the outline of the body, I believe, is unnecessary, in that all the essential investigation concerning the placing of that body should be completed before same is removed; however, under certain circumstances, for example where the person is presumed to be alive and while waiting for an ambulance to remove him, it might be advisable to draw an outline of his position for further study, sketching and pictures.

It should be noted at this time that the investigator should conduct himself well, interrogating and retaining the old witnesses, but with the concept of not creating new ones by conducting an improper and ill-advised type of investigation which might be subject to criticism by those present.

His next step is to write a description of the body, where lying and how lying, describing all visible wounds and bloodstains, where located and, more particularly, the color, size and thickness, amount of drying and shape of the said stains.

The investigator will often find it well rewarding to have a stenographer with him during his investigation so that he may, upon approaching the scene, simply start thinking and talking out loud, having all of his comments noted and later transcribed. This procedure can be of tremendous help in allowing freedom of action, eliminating unnecessary diversion and permitting full description of the entire investigation, plus an accurate, complete and verbatim accounting of everything said and done. (See Forms 23-38.)

INVESTIGATION PROCEDURE

I. Minimum equipment necessary to conduct investigation
    A. Loose leaf notebook
       and
    B. Measuring tape

II. Precepts for investigation
    A. Approach scene with objective, not preconceived opinion
    B. Don't make final evaluation of evidence at first search
       1. Preserve scene
       2. Preserve evidence to prove opinion
       3. Record all pertinent facts
       4. Cross-examine yourself

III. Fundaments of evidence collection (Fig. 1)
    A. Protect against adulteration, contamination and loss
    B. Provide adequate amount of collected material for study and analysis
    C. Keep items separated
    D. Label each item as it is taken
    E. Seal evidence containers
    F. Record chain of evidence, including
       1. Persons in possession of same
       2. Time of transfer
       3. Place of transfer—always obtaining
       4. Receipts for evidence, as transferred to another

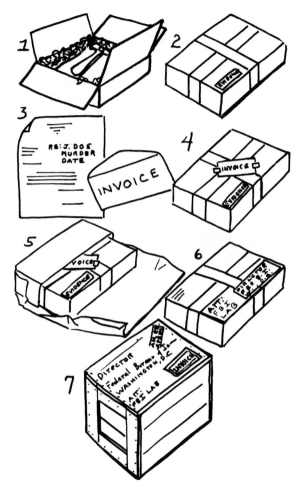

Fig. 1. Evidence should be placed securely in box, sealed and marked, as illustrated above. A copy of transmittal letter should be enclosed in the envelope and marked "Invoice."

IV.   Scope of examination is for
    A.   Comparison
         and/or

B.   Identification
V.   At time of original call, record
    A.   Manner in which call received
    B.   From whom
    C.   Date
      and
    D.   Time
VI.   On arrival on scene, record
    A.   Time
    B.   Place
    C.   Weather conditions
    D.   Persons on scene
      and
    E.   Their information concerning the death
    F.   Survey the body
      1.   Without disturbing or moving
      2.   Just to satisfy self that the subject is dead
      BUT
      3.   If any doubt prevails as to existence of life presume the subject alive and act accordingly
VII.   Preserve the scene by
    A.   Restricting all unnecessary persons from the locale
      AND
    B.   Then conducting a methodical, orderly, air-tight investigation
      1.   Complete description of body
        a.   Where and how lying
        b.   Description of visible wounds
        c.   Description of blood
          (1)   Where located
          (2)   Size

(3) Direction of flow

(4) Color

d. Clothing on subject

    (1) Describe, starting from top to bottom

    (2) Note condition of clothing

e. Jewelry on subject

    Note: If no jewelry, state same

Note: Do not touch or move the body, and describe only what can be seen without the necessity of disturbing the subject

2. Complete description of area (Fig. 2a and Fig. 2b)

a. Note in writing everything observed

b. With free hand, draw the outline of the area

c. Draw permanent fixtures

d. Indicate where body is lying

e. Take accurate measurements

f. Note measurements on the free hand sketch

g. Measure body from permanent fixtures AND

h. Make accurate and permanent diagram at a later time

Note: NEVER substitute photographs for sketch and actual measurements

(See Form 20 for sketch symbols.)

3. Photographs

a. Should be taken by experts

b. In a clockwise direction

c. Starting north

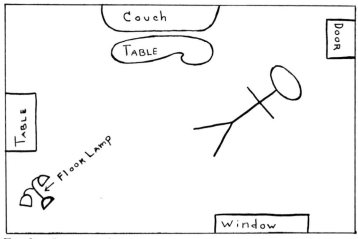

FIG. 2a.   Incorrect sketching.

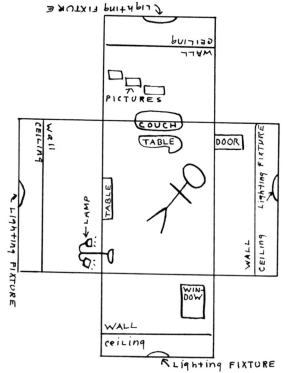

FIG. 2b.   Correct sketching, showing all dimensions.

AND

    d. Taking in everything necessary to describe the locale, the contents and their relationships to the subject

    Note: Body must NOT be touched during any of this time

    Note: Original notes and original diagrams should be retained by investigating officer

VIII. Removing the body to the morgue

    A. Protect the hands by placing bags over same to

      1. Keep them from being contaminated

    AND

      2. Keep people from touching them

    B. Look carefully underneath the body and in the clothing at time of removal to discover bullets or objects which might by lying loose and which might thus fall during removal, thereby being lost

    C. Protect all bloodstains so as not to destroy same

IX. Body at the morgue

    A. Undressing

      1. Clothing should be removed in orderly fashion, without

        a. Cutting or tearing same

        b. Contaminating same, or

        c. Smearing blood or other stains

      2. Garments should be tagged as they are removed, and

      3. They should be hung on hangers and allowed to dry, and

        4. When the clothing is dried it should be
          packaged, sealed and marked

  B. Photographing body
        1. Photos should be taken to show marks
          of violence
        then
        2. Wounds should be cleaned and photos
          again taken of the clean wounds (Fig. 3)

Note: A ruler should be laid alongside the wound
to show size of same

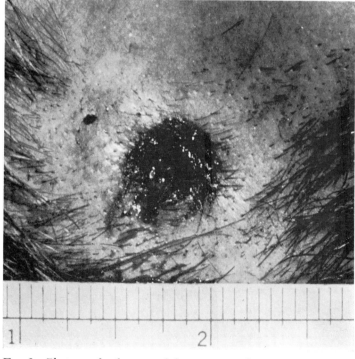

Fig. 3. Photograph of a wound from a vertical position, with ruler
placed alongside wound to indicate actual size of same and to
avoid distortion.

Note: All photographs of wounds should be made from a vertical position so that the picture of the wound will not be distorted

C. Autopsy
   1. Persons present
      a. Pathologist
      b. Police officer
      c. Coroner
      d. All disinterested persons should be barred
   2. Photographs should be made of all the relevant parts of the body
   3. A probe of the wound should be made in photograph to show trajectory and depth
   4. Sections and tissues of the body should be retained by the pathologist for future study and for purposes of anticipating all possible eventualities (Fig. 4.)
   5. Physical evidence, such as bullets, broken pieces of knife blades and the like, should be immediately turned over to the investigating officer by the pathologist

Note: All bodies need not be autopsied
   BUT
   Autopsy should be conducted where there is reason to believe that death was causd by some criminal agent
   EXCEPT
   Where all the investigating officers are certain that the death was caused by suicide

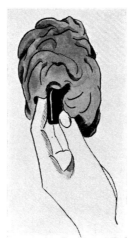

Fig. 4.   Correct manner of recovery of bullet or other object with
fingertips, so as not to mar same.

X.   General notes
   A.   DO NOT
      1.   Smoke on the scene
      2.   Comment to anyone about the guilt or
            innocence of any person
      3.   Be sidetracked by suggestions
      4.   Rely completely on eye witnesses (can
            be unreliable)
      5.   Completely ignore reporters—sometimes
            they can be helpful.

—3—

INVESTIGATOR AND THE PATHOLOGIST

I. Before autopsy
   A. Investigator should inform pathologist of
      1. Description of circumstances of death
      2. Circumstances of the finding of the body
      3. Description of the scene
      4. Statements of witnesses
         BY
         a. Pictures (use of Polaroid pictures is recommended for purposes of immediate study)
         b. Diagrams
         c. Oral description
      Note: Pathologist should be called to the scene where investigator deems it necessary or proper
   B. Investigator should forward to the pathologist pertinent evidence found at scene, such as
      1. Medication
      2. Empty containers
      3. Medicating equipment
      4. Weapons
      5. Samples for laboratory
         AND
      6. All other evidence and clues requiring scientific, medical or technological study

II. Autopsy
- A. The body should be examined and autopsied in as close to natural condition as possible
- B. History of the patient's physical ailments should be discussed, determining any relationship to the death
- C. Pathologist and investigator should converse during the autopsy to create a common understanding of
  1. Connection between prior investigation and autopsy
  2. Mutual understanding as to what is being done
  3. Cause of death
  4. Future investigation and procedure
- D. Objects such as bullets, pieces of weapons and the like should be turned over to the investigator by the pathologist—the pathologist receiving a receipt therefor
- E. Pictures should be taken by the pathologist and/or the investigator as the autopsy progresses

III. Further aid to autopsy by investigator
- A. Protect
  1. Condition of body
  2. Clothing
  3. Blood and other marks
- B. Prevent embalming so as not to destroy some evidences, such as
  1. Some poisons (example: cyanide)
  2. Alcohol
  3. Some evidences of asphyxia
  4. Carbon monoxide
     AND

   5. The draining of the blood from the system

IV. Evidence to be preserved

  A. Blood

  B. Tissues from the various organs of the body

  C. Fingernail clippings

  D. Hair

 Note: Hair should be pulled out by the roots and not cut

  E. Clothing

  F. Where question of rape or molestation, smears

  G. In gunshot wounds, tissue surrounding wounds (to later determine presence or absence of powder burning and depth to where penetrated)

 Note: X-rays are suggested where

  A. Foreign body may be within subject

  B. Where there is a question as to fractures

  C. All teeth, particularly for identification

  D. For presence of fused, melted or otherwise distorted metal objects within the subject (particularly important in electrocution cases, burnings and airplane crashes involving many persons)

  E. Other physical peculiarities or infirmities

V. Autopsy consent (to be used wherever autopsy is desired but legality of same is questionable) (Form 44)

—4—

THE INVESTIGATOR AND THE PUBLIC

It is conceded that the "press" is a very important part of everyday life, and it is also conceded that the "press" owes a duty to the public to report all news that might be educational or of interest; it is also the duty of the investigator, as a servant of the people, to cooperate with the "press" and to preserve harmony and good relationship with same, reporting to it all news which might be of interest, provided, however, that the investigator does not reveal information which might jeopardize the case, or information which might not necessarily be true or accurate.

An investigator should be very careful to divulge only those facts of which he is certain, and only those facts which will not hamper later investigation nor injure an innocent party unnecessarily.

Firstly, the investigator should not divulge an alleged identity of a person, but should wait until such time as that person has been definitely identified by the proper authorities and by a close relative or friend. He should likewise not divulge the alleged cause of death until such time that the pathologist has definitely determined same after an examination or autopsy. He should not theorize on the weapon or weapons used or on the effects of same until there is no doubt as to the certainty of this fact. He should not divulge any particulars of the death until such time that his superiors or the coroner's office determine which step or steps should be taken to complete the investigation. He should not allow the reporters to conduct

their own private investigation and thereafter report alleged clues that might be later proven to be untrue, or
that might jeopardize the investigation. He should not
reveal any information until such time as his superiors or
the coroner's office are first informed of same. He should
not reveal the name of the deceased until such time that
the relatives are informed of the death by the proper
officials.

He should treat the "press" with courtesy and consideration and should reveal definite and accurate information
after consent to do so is given by either his superiors or by
the coroner's office. He should be certain of his facts before he states them and should carefully consider each and
every statement before he utters it. He should decline
revealing of conjectures or theories. He should state only
what he saw, heard or observed, and should not hazard a
guess as to possible indictments or convictions or legal
or medical conclusions.

Likewise, it is the duty of the "press," as a reporter of
the people, to cooperate with the authorities and to forego
the possibility of a bloodthirsty headline for a humane,
true, accurate story which would not unduly harm an
innocent person, mislead the public, hamper the investigation of a case, or create a panic.

It is also the duty of the officer and of the "press" to
utilize this medium of publicity to help in investigation
wherever possible, and, more particularly, to help trace
unidentified persons.

Officials owe a duty to the public to divulge noteworthy
news, and the "press" owes a duty to the public to see that
it gets that news accurately and as soon as possible, but
the "press" also owes a duty both to the public and to the
investigating authorities to utilize this medium in such a
manner as to inform the public as soon as possible, and as

fully as possible, and, at the same time, serve that public by aiding the officials in their conducting of the investigation, and in not hampering same.

The investigator should also deal humanely and diplomatically with the bereaved family of the deceased. He should realize their loss and should take cognizance of the fact that the sudden shock of the news of a death of one close to them might affect their ability to reason properly, and might make them a little nervous and sharp.

He should realize their concerns and their doubts and should treat them accordingly.

He should also call for medical help when they seem in shock and should call for religious help to aid in healing their mental and moral wounds.

It is not only his duty to investigate a case and find the guilty person or persons, but also to protect not only the safety but the health and mind of fellow human beings (Fig. 5).

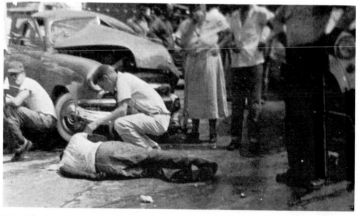

Fig. 5. Incorrect manner to investigate a scene; spectators and onlookers should be politely but firmly removed from the scene proper.

—5—

REPORT WRITING

I. Purpose
- A. To provide permanent record of information obtained by investigation
- B. To communicate information obtained
- C. To provide other investigators with a basis for continuation of investigation
- D. To enable reviewing officers to determine whether the investigation is being properly developed
- E. To keep all officials abreast of current investigations
- F. To assist officials in evaluating case at hand
- G. To be used in preparation of case for prosecution

II. Source of the report
- A. The immediate source of information should be embodied in the report
- B. Later report at headquarters should
  1. Condense information
  2. Clarify information
  3. Arrange notes

III. Notebook
- A. Should be loose leaf
  1. Should be used only for information relative to police work
  2. Should not have miscellaneous scribblings
  3. Should not contain any "doodling".

B. Notes referring to particular case should be kept together in the notebook

C. In making notes of interviews with separate persons, keep notes of each individual on separate pages

D. Be accurate as to time, dates and places

E. Record all weather conditions accurately

F. Do not erase, but draw one line through any mistake

G. In recording an interview, attempt to use exact words, especially in key sentences, as much as possible

H. Do not use scrap paper in making notes

IV. Questions to be answered

A. WHAT
What happened?

B. WHEN
1. When was it discovered?
2. When was the officer notified

C. WHERE
1. Where did it occur?
2. Where were persons connected with the investigation?
3. Where were objects connected with the investigation

D. HOW
1. How was the event accomplished?
2. How did the event take place?

E. WHY
1. Why did it happen?
2. Events taking place immediately preceding the offense?

F. WHO
    1. Who were the persons concerned?
    2. Their names, ages, residence, description, etcetera?

IV. Most important things in writing notes are clarity, conciseness and simplicity, attempting to avoid slang and bad English and very carefully watching spelling
(See Forms 23-38)

—6—

INTERROGATION

As soon as the investigating officers have completed their search, sketching, photographing and preliminary investigation, their attention should next be directed to the persons on the premises and other possible witnesses. Before the body is removed, at least one of these people should be called upon to identify the victim.

It is recommended that at least two officers be present during the interrogation of witnesses, so that one may corroborate the statement of the other at a later time, should the witness decide to change his story or deny any part of the said statement.

Witnesses should be questioned separately, and no other witnesses should be present in the room at the time while the one witness is telling his story; as a matter of fact, if there are a number of persons to be questioned, no one witness, even after telling his story, should be allowed to mingle with those who have not yet told their story, for the obvious reason that he could influence the testimony of those who come after him.

Before actually interrogating a witness, the officer should do his utmost to put the witness at ease, and attempt to gain his respect and confidence. He should extend his sympathy for the loss of his loved one, comment briefly upon the misfortune suffered by the victim, and have a short general conversation with the witness. He should then begin his questioning with "Will you please state your full name?" and should then inquire as to what is known as the "full pedigree" of the witness, which pedigree includes the witness' name, date of birth, address, marital status, number of children, employment, place of birth and all other matters which will give the officer an insight as to his life history and background, and which will make it easier at a later time to check the record of the witness, and his credibility, character and reputation, if that becomes necessary.

He should then determine the relationship between the witness and the victim, the length of their acquaintanceship, the type of relationship, e.g., how intimate the relationship was. By doing this he can find out many facts concerning the life of the victim and determine just how much the witness may have known of the victim's life, and how much the victim may have confided in the witness. He can thusly "dig" and locate many important clues and may thereby find the treasure of any violent death, the motive.

The witness should then be interrogated as to his knowledge of the victim's background and as to anything that might have happened within a reasonable time prior to the death of the victim, which could have some bearing upon that death, or might bear upon the motive.

The witness should then be very carefully and methodically questioned about all events which happened a reasonable time prior to the death of the victim, and particularly on the day of the death. Questioning should then dwell upon the death itself, and upon what he saw or observed immediately preceding, during and following the death, or as soon thereafter as the death was discovered.

The witness should then be allowed to express himself upon any observations or suspicions that he might have, and then should be questioned as to anything that he heard anybody else say prior to, at the time of, or after the death of the victim, which might have a bearing upon that death.

It is very important that the officer calmly question the witness and ask questions which the witness may answer himself instead of pretending to lead the witness. It is also important that the witness be allowed to answer these questions in his own words, and then be called upon to explain his answers as fully as possible. A witness who talks freely and who is allowed to talk as much as he desires is the one who will give the most information both intentionally and unintentionally.

Before, during and after the interrogation of the witnesses, the officer should attempt to be as polite as possible, using in effect "sugar" or "honey" to put his witness at ease, and to put him in the mood and frame of mind to talk freely. This is done not only because it is the duty and obligation of the officer to conduct himself as a gentleman, but with the thought that a carefree and non-belligerent tongue is the best witness as far as questioning is concerned, and with the thought that a mind at ease is the best thinking mind as far as accurate memory is concerned.

Once the questioning officer has determined that the interrogation could conceivably be relevant in the investigation of the death, he should at that time take down in writing the full statement of the witness, dating the statement, and having it signed, with each page and all corrections being initialed. No erasures should be used, but rather corrections should be marked through with one line.

At that point, the officers should witness the signature and sign as witnesses under the signature, and it is suggested that where there is a suspicion that the witness may be later implicated in the crime that he is immediately rushed to headquarters where he might make a second statement that can be taken down more fully in shorthand and completely transcribed.

To eliminate the possibility of a later repudiation of the statement by the witness and to eliminate his later accusation that duress or force had been used, it is suggested that there always be at least two officers present at the time that the interrogation is being made.

On the spot questioning and interrogation is very important not only in determining the immediate facts that may help in that investigation, but also in securing a complete, voluntary and true story while the facts and circumstances are still fresh in the witness' mind, and before he has time to contemplate over a more advantageous and distorted statement. It has also been found that a statement is much more easily secured in the immediate surroundings than in the confines of a jail or police headquarters.

Note: A confession by a defendant is admissible at a later trial after the establishment of a corpus delicti by the State and upon showing that the confession was not forced by duress or other illegal or devious manners. A statement by one other than the defendant is admissible at a later time only if that statement was made in the presence of the defendant; otherwise, the statement is hearsay evidence, and is not admissible.

—7—

CONFESSIONS

I. Admissibility
   A. Must be voluntary
   B. Must be without duress or force
   C. Must be without the promise of any immunity
   D. Must be after advising the subject of his Constitutional privilege to refuse to testify (in some jurisdictions, this step is not necessary)
   E. In some jurisdictions, must be in writing

II. *DO NOT*
   A. Use physical abuse or threat of abuse
   B. Question over a persistent and prolonged period of time
   C. Question in the presence of many persons
   D. Make promises to secure a false confession
   E. Merge into one confession statements taken on several crimes

III. If more than one person is involved
   A. Question separately
   B. Keep separated in different rooms while waiting to be questioned

IV. On written statements or confessions
   A. Have subject initial or sign every page
   B. Do not erase
   C. Have subject initial every error
   D. As closely as possible quote subject verbatim

34

E. Have signatures and initials of subject witnessed by at least one other party

F. Have only one person interrogate

G. Record time and place of interrogation

H. Have subject sign under certification similar to the following

I have read the above statement given to officers
_____and_____, of
my own free will and accord and without the promise of
any immunity or extra favors and without any duress or
force, and after having been told of my Constitutional
privileges as an American Citizen to refuse to testify,
and I find that the above statement is true according
to my best knowledge and belief.

In Witness Whereof, I set my hand at_____
(address) in the County of_____,
this_____day of_____, 19_____.

_____
(Full name)

_____
_____
(Witnesses)

V. Scene

A. Have subject reconstruct scene in presence of witnesses

B. Take pictures of relevant positions and demonstrations

C. Have subject identify weapons used

D. Have subject initial weapons

—8—

DYING DECLARATIONS

SYNOPSIS

At times an officer may arrive on a call and it is apparent to him that the subject will probably die in a matter of moments. In the time between the actual arrival of the officer and the later arrival of a physician or ambulance, it is sometimes possible for the officer to secure a statement from that person, which statement may later prove to be important in determining whether or not a crime did exist and in investigating the circumstances surrounding that crime.

One of these types of statements is termed a "dying declaration." A dying declaration is a statement that is made by a victim who believes that he is dying and who believes that there is no hope of recovery. This statement or declaration must concern the cause of his injury or his death, and as such is admissible at a trial dealing with the death of that particular individual. The fact that the individual did not die after making such a declaration does not negate the validity of this declaration so long as the person did believe that he was about to die and had no hope of recovery at the time.

In taking a dying declaration, the officer should first question the subject to determine whether he is in a proper state of mind to realize what he is saying and to recall the facts that have occurred. The person usually makes the declaration orally; however, it is suggested that notes be made by the officer during the time that the declaration is being given, and that these notes be more fully developed as soon as possible thereafter, being careful to use the actual words of the subject as much as possible.

A dying declaration should commence with the name of the victim, his address, the fact that he believes that he is about to die and has no chance of recovery, the fact that he recalls what happened, the approximate date and the approximate time of the statement itself, and finally the statement.

The officer should try, if possible, to write the complete statement and have the subject sign it, after reading it to the subject or having him read it himself if he is physically able to do so.

It is very important if the subject dies, and after his death, that he be identified by the police and by relatives or close friends as the one who made the declaration. The presence of at least two persons during all of this procedure is desirable but not essential.

Another type of statement from a dying person is the confession, and the same procedure as outlined above should be followed in this case, except that it is not necessary for the person to be certain that he is going to die to make the confession valid and admissible in court as evidence.

It is recommended that dying declarations or confessions be written in ink or typed, and that no erasures be made. In the event of a mistake, the word or words should be lined out (one line) and initialed.

DYING DECLARATION

I. General
   One of the few types of hearsay evidence admissible for the purpose of incriminating and convicting another person

II. Elements
   A. Person must believe he is going to die
      AND
      must have lost all hope of recovery
   B. His statement should refer only to
      1. Manner
      2. Circumstances
         and
      3. Identification of persons responsible for
         Ultimate death
   C. He must die
   D. This statement can be used only in the trial for death of declarant

III. Statement may be oral or written, but if feasible
   A. Reduce to writing
   B. Have declarant sign or make mark
   C. Have witnesses present

IV. Be on guard to determine
   A. Whether the witness is competent
   B. Would he wish to mislead the interrogator
   C. Is he under influence of drugs or in shock
   D. Does physical evidence negate his dying declaration

E. Are these statements facts of which he has personal knowledge, or are they merely opinions of which he is surmising

Note: Attempt to have witness identify accused

Note: Write in ink—do *not* erase. If a mistake is made, draw one line through a word, initial and write substitute word

Note: If the declarant can recognize the weapon, have him mark same

—9—

PHOTOGRAPHS
SYNOPSIS

Before the touching or removing of the body or any possible evidence on the scene, that entire scene should be studied, sketched and photographed. The photographs should be taken with the purpose of revealing and reproducing the scene in as close and clear detail as is possible under the circumstances, keeping in mind that this photographing is effectual not only as possible evidence in describing what was being observed, but also as a later memory refresher. Pictures should also be taken with the thought of "blowing them up" and studying them at a later time as an additional and exacting "eye." The methodical and complete studying of a normal or "blown up" photograph will oftentimes reveal small but very important particles of evidence that can conceivably be missed by the human searching eye.

Firstly, photographs should be taken of the outside of the house, starting at the front door and proceeding in a clockwise direction completely around the house; these pictures should show the general view of the outside of the house, the surrounding grounds and the particulars of the house itself.

Then pictures should be taken of the rooms of the house, being careful to avoid distortion and to take the photographs in such a manner as to tell a story. In order to keep continuity, it is recommended that the pictures be taken in a clockwise direction, commencing with the camera facing north. Whenever a picture is taken of any particular object in more than one direction, the photographer should take the group of pictures at approximately the same angle and from approximately the same distance; then he may take pictures from whatever other angles and distances he thinks are necessary under the circumstances.

In the absence of proper camera equipment, and in the desire to take pictures of a small object, the photographer should be extremely careful not to sacrifice clearness in order to get a closer and larger view of the object, keeping in mind that a smaller and clearer picture can at a later time be "blown up," whereas a blurred close-up cannot be corrected.

Pictures should then be taken of the body itself from various angles for the purpose of identification and demonstration of clues, position, facial expressions, limbs, flow of blood, excretion from the body, together with the relationship of that body to blood spots, the room generally, location of weapons and other evidence, upset or disturbed furniture, and the like. This group of pictures is especially important to aid in the determination of the cause of death, the proving or disproving of any crime, and a later reconstruction of the circumstances surrounding the death.

In taking these pictures, the photographer must be careful and methodical, firstly determining what facts need to be shown, how they should be shown and the best manner of reproducing them, before actually taking any photographs. Finally, he should not be "stingy" in the number of pictures he takes, but should realize that it is far more practical to disregard unnecessary reproductions than to have to regret the lack of an all important one.

PHOTOGRAPHS

I. Purpose
   A. To explain how the crime took place
   B. To show all possible elements of the crime
   C. To show the scene from all angles
   D. To show evidence and its location
   E. For study purposes for clues that may have been overlooked by the human eye

II. Indoor scenes should include
   A. House and grounds on which building located
   B. Room where body was found
   C. Adjoining rooms
   D. Entry and exit points
   E. Places of concealment
   F. Evidences of struggle
   G. Situation immediately before occurrence (drinking glasses, food, lighting, etcetera)
   H. Anything unusual or unnatural
   I. Evidence (such as blood marks, fingerprints, broken glass, pills, etcetera)

III. Outdoor scene should include (Fig. 6)
   A. Objects which will identify location
   B. Impressions in the ground (tire marks, shoe marks, etcetera)
   C. Effect on foliage (bent grass blades, broken branches, etcetera)

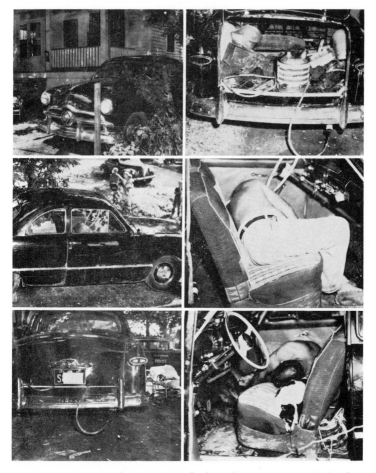

Fig. 6. A group of pictures which tell a story and further identifies automobile and location.

D. Signs of struggle
E. Signs of whether the body was moved
F. Area underneath body as compared to area adjoining body

IV. Hanging
    A. Rafter or roof to which ligature is tied
    B. Type of knot
    C. Manner in which applied to neck
    D. Knot about neck
    E. Facial features
        1. Cyanosis
        2. Condition of tongue
        3. Aspiration
    F. Relation of feet to ground
        1. Whether touching
        2. If above ground, how far above
    G. Ground immediately beneath feet
    H. Stepping-off point
    I. Signs of struggle
    J. Place from which ligature was taken or cut

V. Shooting (Fig. 7 and Fig. 8)
    A. Entrance wound
    B. Exit wound
    C. Powder burns
    D. Position of subject
    E. Firearm itself
    F. Possible trajectories
    G. Ejected cartridges
    H. Penetrating slugs
    I. Places in building itself where bullet may have struck
    J. Points of ricochet
    K. Picture illustrating probable place from where bullet was fired and angle of travel

VI. Electrocution
    A. Entrance marks on bodies

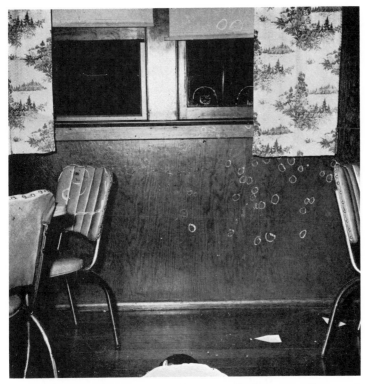

FIG. 7 Photograph showing disbursing of shotgun pellets and pointers illustrating location of other clues on the floor.

B. Exit marks on bodies
C. Electrical equipment involved
D. Place where body probably ground
E. Of over-all scene to reconstruct what the deceased was doing at time of shock

VII. Drowning
A. Face of subject
1. To show whether foam coming from mouth

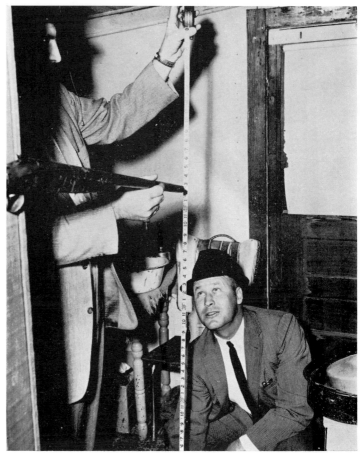

Fig. 8. Reconstruction of a scene, showing location of weapon
and trajectory.

            2. To show whether mouth was open or
closed

            3. To show possible cyanosis in face

    B.   Hands

            1. To show cadavaric spasm to determine
whether or not subject was grabbing for
anything

      2. To determine whether hands were tied

   C. Entire body

      1. To show bruises

      2. To show anything peculiar or suspicious

   D. Clothing

      1. To determine possibility of struggle

VIII. Fires

   A. Area of origin

   B. Direction of spread of fire

   C. Type of fire

   D. Arrangements of all apertures (doors and windows)

   E. Position of bodies

   F. Of over-all scene to reconstruct what deceased was doing at time of fire

IX. DO NOT

   A. Allow investigators to be photographed on scene

   B. Rely on photographs without accompanying sketches

   C. Be ignorant of your jurisdiction (some states permit colored photographs to be entered into evidence whereas others do not)

X. Cameras

   A. Polaroid

      1. To have picture for immediate reference

      2. To have picture to convey to morgue with body to reconstruct scene for pathologist

   B. Black and white

   C. Colored

      1. To be able to reconstruct scene accurately as to colors and shades

        2. To be able to portray on a screen for detailed study

    D. Movies

        1. To photograph scene entailing abnormally large area (such as disasters)

        2. To reproduce confessions or statements and to use same to corroborate them

XI. Pictures should be marked in back, to state

    A. Time taken

    B. Date taken

    C. Place taken

    D. Name of photographer

    E. Direction from which taken

    F. Distance from which taken

    G. Type of camera used

    H. Lens opening

    I. Type of lens

(Form 19)

—10—

TRANSPORTATION OF BODIES

Careful moving and transporting of the body of a victim is very important so as not to destroy any evidence that might later be discovered under the careful scrutiny of experts, pathologists and medical technologists. Likewise, in moving a body, one should be very careful not to destroy any evidence that may lie underneath or be in any way covered by the corpse.

The body should be moved under the direction and supervision of the coroner and/or officer at the scene. In lifting the body, as much help should be utilized as may be needed to raise the body directly off the surface without wrinkling the clothes, smearing the blood or other stains, or changing or damaging any kind of evidence or clues that might lie underneath the body. Whenever possible, the body should be placed upon a litter in approximately the same position in which it was found, and that body tied down so that there will be no movement during the transportation of same.

Any objects which may be associated with the body should be moved at the same time, so that they might be examined in the morgue and their relationship to the death established.

Any soft tissues, pieces of bone, pieces of skull, pieces of skin or other remains of the body that have become disarticulated from the body should be carefully wrapped and transported in such a way as to eliminate the possibility of its falling apart or becoming further distorted.

No possessions or personal belongings should be removed from the subject's body, except under the direction of the coroner or his pathologist.

Upon arrival at the morgue, the same care should be taken in transferring the body from the wagon to the slab. The driver and his helper should remain with the body and its accompanying parts until the person in charge of the morgue has arrived and has made note of and taken charge of the same.

Careful transportation of a victim is a very important element of investigation and examination, and the transporter should consider himself an important trustee in the protection and preservation of whatever evidence might exist.

(See Form 38—Report to Accompany Body to Morgue.)

—11—

COLLECTION, HANDLING AND SHIPPING
OF EVIDENCE

SYNOPSIS

As important, and sometimes even more important, and certainly more effective in front of a jury, is the presentation of evidence which establishes a corpus delicti and points a finger at the accused.

Therefore, one of the main elements of an investigation is the recognition, collection, interpretation and presentation of evidence—always preserving links in a chain among those who have handled the evidence, so that final testimony will indicate in whose possession this evidence was, how it was examined, the fact that it was not mutilated or contaminated, and finally that it was the same bit of evidence originally found at the scene.

This section deals with the collection of some evidence, but in an over-all picture, it is essential for the investigator to realize the standards that are necessary for the said collection, same being: (1) the evidence itself; (2) desired quantity; (3) manner of submission to laboratory or expert; and (4) required control of evidence for comparison.

Packaging of evidence, in the main, requires only good common sense as to what will best protect that article, keeping in mind that each bit of evidence should be marked, separately packaged, noted on the report where the evidence was marked and how packaged, the chain of evidence, and delivering it to a laboratory or experts as soon as possible.

The investigator should describe whatever changes might occur in the nature of the evidence, further explaining why and how the same occurred.

The investigator's job is not completed when the evidence is merely packaged and taken to a laboratory. In order to permit the technician to obtain from the evidence the maximum in clues and information, this investigator should advise the said technician of all the facts obtained in the case and what to look for.

Finally, the evidence is usually presented in Court, and its presentation depends, to a great extent, on the skill of the investigator; therefore, before presenting this evidence in Court the investigator should: (1) review the material and the evidence; (2) consult with others on the case; (3) review the case file; and (4) recollect where and how each piece was marked.

(Form 39—Evidence Collection.)

(Form 40—Receipts for Evidence.)

COLLECTION, HANDLING AND SHIPPING
OF EVIDENCE

I. Definition
  A. To prove or disprove a matter
     AND
  B. To influence belief or disbelief of persons at
     1. The investigation
        AND
     2. At the trial

II. Evidence is presented through
  A. Verbal recounting
     AND/OR
  B. Physical objects
     BUT
  C. Whether by verbal accounting or physical object must be presented by and through witnesses

III. Evidence must be
  A. Legally obtained
  B. Legally handled
  C. Properly presented before the Court and a Jury
     AND
  D. Fully explored
  E. Completely protected
  F. Properly identified
  G. Adequately described
     AND, therefore

      H.   Material which may become evidence must be
- 1. Recognized immediately
  - a. Of its value
    - AND
  - b. Its potential use in the case

IV. The scene must be recorded and fully explored by
- A. Pictures
- B. Sketches
- C. Notes
- D. Systematic search of the scene (in a clockwise direction)
  - AND
- E. Obtaining relevant information to go with the evidence

V. Check list of investigation of home
- A. Stairs, passages, entries to scene, streets, yards and neighborhood
- B. Outer doors—bolted, locks, marks of breaking in
- C. Waste basket or dust bins
- D. Windows
- E. Letter box (date of mail)
- F. Papers, milk, etc. (date)
- G. Inside door — locked, bolted — on what side key
- H. Closets — position of clothing, etcetera
- I. Lighting — which lights on or off
- J. Heating condition
- K. Smell
- L. Clocks and watches
- M. Ash trays
- N. Containers and bottles

O. Kitchen, bathroom (towels, sinks, commodes, etcetera)
P. Damages
Q. Garments
R. Notes, letters, books
S. Hanging—source of rope
Note: DO NOT smoke, light or throw away matches, dispose of gum wrappers or anything of the like that might be confused with evidence on the scene

VI. Check list concerning deceased (Fig. 9)
A. Name, age, sex, nationality, occupation

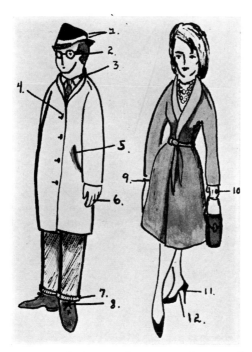

FIG. 9. Locations in clothing to be examined in search for small clues such as hairs, dust, fibers and the like.

    B.   Residence and business addresses

    C.   Names, addresses and phone numbers of all members of family and relatives

    D.   Lodges and clubs

    E.   Character

    F.   Friends—names

    G.   Lawyer, doctor, dentist, minister, business associates

    H.   Religious beliefs

    I.   Education

    J.   Disposition, health and habits

    K.   Past addresses

    L.   Where he was at least 48 hours before death

    M.   With whom he talked and visited, what said, where headed

    N.   What doing just before killed

    O.   What doing at time killed

    P.   Immediate plans

    Q.   Insurance

    R.   Own any weapons—carry them

    S.   Apparent cause of death

    T.   Description

    U.   Apparel

    V.   Possessions and jewelry on person

    W.   Last person to see him alive (where, when, etcetera)

VII.   Collection and preservation of evidence (Fig. 10)

    A.   Tools

        1. Take all

        2. Wrap in cotton or paper

        3. Place tool at the bottom of a strong cardboard carton

        4. Punch holes through the bottom of the carton around the edge of the tools

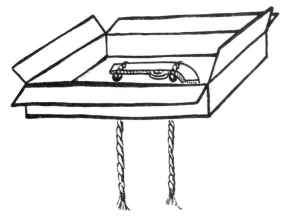

Fig. 10. Correct manner to package guns, knives, tools and other objects for preservation of fingerprints, dirt, fibers, blood and other clues that might be thereon. Note holes cut in bottom of box and string used to tie object to keep it from rubbing against surface.

       5. Tie tools in place
       6. Objects bearing tool marks should be so packed as to protect them from friction or scratching

  B. Documents (example: checks, letters, handwriting, typewriting, erasures, ink, etcetera)
       1. Handle document as little as possible
       2. Do not fold or otherwise crease
       3. Place in large envelope
       4. Further protect with stiff cardboard, so that it will not bend
       5. For comparison, obtain
          a. Samples of suspect's writing
          b. Sheets of paper for comparison
          c. Samples of typewriting
          d. Erasers

      e. Have suspect write 10 to 20 copies on separate sheets of paper at various spots for comparison

C.   Soil

    1. Prevent sample from becoming contaminated with other soil

    2. If soil is adhering to some other objects, such as clothing, shoes and the like

        a. Leave the soil attached to the object

        b. Place in a clean box lined with paper

    3. If soil is free from other objects

        a. Obtain representative sample of soil

        b. Place in a clean glass container
           OR

        c. In a druggist fold
           OR

        d. Tightly sealed box

    4. For comparison obtain

        a. Clothing from suspect
           OR

        b. Soil samples

  Note: Do not dig into ground to get sample, but take from surface

  Note: Do not pull up grass or weeds to get soil off the roots

D.   Clothing

    1. Take all

    2. If wet, hang to dry

    3. Pack only one garment to a box, protecting

        a. Stains

        b. Dust

      c. Other objects adhering to clothing

    Note: If clothes are submitted for powder burning determination, place a clean sheet of white paper on either side of cloth in the region of the bullet hole

E. Wire
1. Obtain all
2. Wrap in paper and place rigidly in a box
3. Obtain approximately 2 feet of comparison wire

F. Glass (Fig. 11)
1. Obtain all
2. Wrap each piece in cotton or soft paper, protecting stains and prints
3. Place rigidly in a box
   AND
4. Obtain any glass suspected of being identical or from which evidence may have come

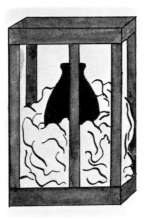

FIG. 11. Packaging of bottles and other glass. Note paper or cotton between that and wooden box to keep from breaking or becoming contaminated.

G. Paint stains
1. Take all
2. Scrape off or cut out portion of material with stain
3. Place in a clean box
4. Obtain paint scrapings from objects necessary for comparison
AND
5. If wet, place in glass jar
H. Fibers
1. Take all
2. Place in small pill-box or druggist fold (Fig. 12)

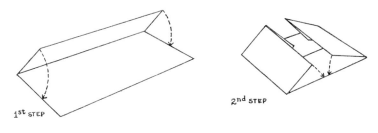

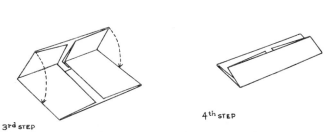

FIG. 12. Illustration indicating druggist's or jeweler's fold—to be used for packaging of fibers, hairs and the like.

AND
3. Obtain samples from which suspected fibers may have come

I. Fingernail scrapings for soil, dust, hair, fibers, blood, skin
1. Scraping from each fingernail should be wrapped separately
2. Should be placed in pill-box or test tube
3. Should be specifically labeled to show from which finger obtained

J. Plaster cast (Figs. 13, a and b)

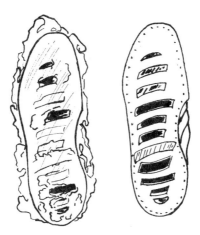

FIG. 13a. Illustration indicating footmarks in mud and clarity of plaster cast made from same.

1. Photograph
   a. Place a ruler close to the impression
   b. Take photo from directly above impression
2. Remove extraneous material from impression
3. Place metal frame around impression; allow 1″ margin and about 1½″ deep

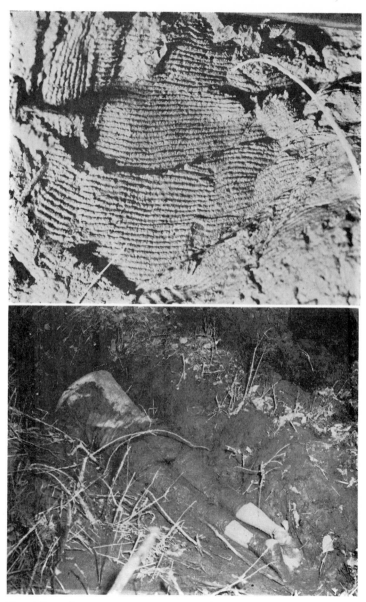

Fig. 13b. Plaster paris cast showing fabrics of sweater and position of subject in mud.

4. Use twigs or wires to re-enforce material
5. Mix plaster
   a. Make it creamy
      AND
   b. Eliminate all lumps
6. Pour quickly into frame approximately ½″ in depth
7. Place re-enforcing wires or twigs
8. Add balance of plaster

Note: If impression is dusty or dirty, first coat layer with quick drying shellac or the like, with a very, very thin coat

(Fig. 14)

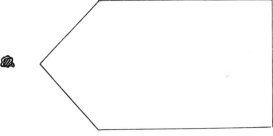

FIG. 14. Illustration indicating the cutting of a small piece of paper pointing to a small clue, to be photographed before removed.

—12—

COURT APPEARANCE

I. Preparation for Court
   A. Collection of all reports in one file
      1. Offense report
      2. Follow-up report
      3. Officer's statements
      4. Evidence receipts
      5. Photographs
      6. Sketches
      7. Working notes
      8. Correspondence
      9. Witnesses' statements
      10. Suspect's statements
      11. Autopsy report
      12. List of physical evidence
         a. Importance of each item
         b. Recovered by whom and where
         c. How marked
         d. Where marked
         e. By whom
   B. State's witnesses
      1. Investigating officers
      2. Coroner or deputies
      3. Pathologist
      4. Medical technologist
      5. Ambulance drivers
      6. Hospital physicians
      7. Defendant

     8. Witnessses
     9. Expert witnesses
    10. Relatives and friends of deceased
    11. Relatives and friends of defendant

II. Conduct of testifying investigator
- A. Dress conservatively
- B. Sit erect
- C. Be polite and gentlemanly
- D. Listen carefully to each question (if question is not understood, ask attorney to repeat or explain)
- E. Answer only question asked (do not volunteer information)
- F. Wherever possible just answer "yes" or "no"
- G. Look directly at attorney or jury when answering questions.
- H. If mistake is made, admit same immediately and make correction
- I. If memory is unclear, state so
- J. Control your temper, especially with defense lawyers (do not regard them as an enemy)
- K. When attorney makes an objection, do not state anything until the Court has made its ruling
- L. Do not make any statements about case in front of other witnesses or jurors while waiting to be called
- M. Tell the truth, even when you think it may prove defendant's innocence
- N. Notebook
  1. Should contain only notes relating to case

2. Should not contain any "doodling" or scribbling
3. Should contain no personal comments or suppositions

—13—

IDENTIFICATION OF DECEASED
SYNOPSIS

For conviction in a criminal trial, two elements of proof are necessary: firstly, that the act itself was committed, and, secondly, that it was done by the person charged or indicted. The first of the necessary proofs is termed corpus delicti, which literally means the body of the offense or crime. The corpus delicti, or the offense itself, is to be distinguished from the performance of the act by a person. In the case of a homicide, the corpus delicti is proof that a person has died by violence and not merely that he has died.

The corpus delicti, under very rare circumstances, can be proven by circumstantial evidence, provided that the evidence is believed by the jury beyond a reasonable doubt. Proof of this nature might conceivably be necessary in the case of a drowning when the body has not been recovered, or of a burning where the ashes have been disposed of. It is recommended that where it might be necessary to prove a corpus delicti by circumstantial evidence, all witnesses and possible culprits be questioned immediately as to when the deceased was last seen and as to any evidence that might throw a presumptive light upon his disappearance.

Definite identification of the dead body is also an important factor in the establishment of corpus delicti. Although this cannot be established by the photographs themselves, they are very useful, and should be taken to accomplish the following purposes: to show clothes, general appearance, size, physical characteristics (showing of physical characteristics should be done by photographs taken after the body is cleaned and put in as natural a state as possible), and other features and factors about the deceased. Although there is a tendency among courts not to permit colored photographs, it is believed that they are more acceptable for the purposes of identification than are black and white ones. In the use of photographs for identification, mirrors and angle shots may be used, so that several views of the deceased can be shown at one time.

These photographs should firstly be taken at the scene and supplemented by others taken at the morgue, the latter being used for the purpose of showing the deceased in a clear or more natural condition.

X-rays should also be taken to show the teeth, bone structure, wounds, possible former injuries and the like. Description of the body itself should indicate sex, measurements of the body, weight, scars, type and color of hair, type and color of eyes, shape of nose, mouth, shape of head and face, fingerprints, physical condition, type of hands, size of clothes and shoes, complexion, teeth, approximate age, blood types, and other general matters such as the probable occupation, social status, background as shown by his clothing, and general appearance.

Wearing apparel should be described in detail, listing all of the articles worn, their size, brand name, place of purchase, cleaning marks, laundry marks and other relevant information, and should further include the general appearance, stained marks of the clothes, etcetera. It should also be known whether there is any indication that the victim wore glasses at or prior to the time he was found.

Identification for its own purpose and for purposes of corpus delicti is an essential factor, and even though the subject has been long dead and his body appearance altered by burning or the elements, modern science goes a long way in proving his identity. A skeleton itself can tell a very definite story. Through some of its bones or its teeth, it is often possible to determine and/or establish identification. The sex of the subject can usually be determined by the examination of the skull, the hip bones and the sacrum of the skeleton. By the presence of even one hair in the skull of the skeleton, one may be able to determine his age, sex and race. Height, approximate size and age are other factors that can be revealed through the bones' structure and developments.

The shape of the skull may be as informative as fingerprints in identifying the victim; in fact, there is a move among scientific law enforcement officials to discard fingerprints and use skull measurements and skull contour to establish identity. No matter how little of the skeleton is left or how badly it is mutilated, it is important in identification purposes, and should be carefully removed and handled without destroying, breaking or losing any portion, so that it may be studied in the morgue by pathologists and anthropologists.

By the same token, even ashes, where there is a possibility the subject may have been burned to death, should be carefully removed and placed in a large box to be examined NOT ON THE SCENE but in the confines of the morgue and laboratory by the expert.

(Form 32—Report of Missing Person.)

(Form 33—General Physical Appearance Report.)

IDENTIFICATION OF DECEASED

I. Definite identification of deceased is necessary for
    A.   Insurance purposes
    B.   Relatives
    C.   To establish a corpus delicti
II. Check list
    A.   General (Fig. 15)
        1. Age (through anatomy, teeth, patholog-
            ical changes, skin, etcetera)

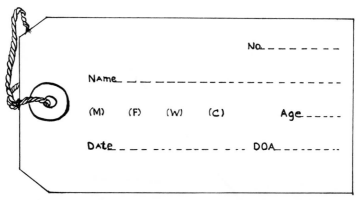

Fig. 15. Identification tag to be tied on wrist, ankle or toe of deceased.

        2. Sex
        3. Height
        4. Weight (do not over-estimate because of
            bloating)
        5. Fingerprints
        6. Race

7. Blood groups—serology
8. Eyes (color, shape, spectacles, etcetera)
9. Nose (shape, size)
10. Teeth (shape, color, notchings, gaps, fillings, dentures, cavities, etcetera)
11. Scars (Fig. 16)
12. Tonsils, appendix, gall bladder, etcetera —present or removed
13. Ears (shape, deformities, size, closeness to head)
14. Hair (color, texture, quantity, dye, comparison)
15. Mouth (shape, lips, scars, etcetera)
16. Skin (color, texture, etcetera)

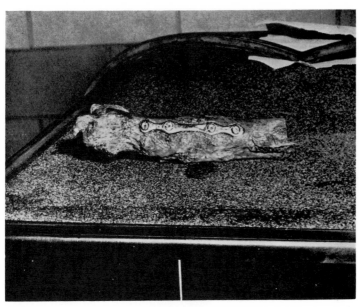

Fig. 16. Identification through operative plate.

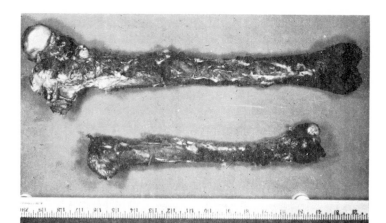

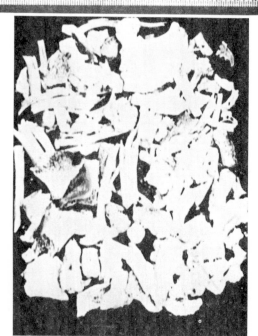

Fig. 17. Bones and teeth recovered from fire; determination of apparent age and physical characteristics by these remains.

17. Head (shape, measurements, anatomy)
18. Special peculiarities (scars, moles, tatooing, bluing, etcetera)
19. Trunk (size, shape, etcetera)
20. Limbs (Fig. 17)
    a. Size of arms, legs, hands, feet
    b. Occupational marks
    c. Condition of skin and nails
    d. Social status—nicotine stains
21. Pathological changes
    a. Special conditions—heart, etcetera
    b. Operative conditions
    c. Accidents
    d. Circumcised
22. Clothing (size, laundry marks, nature, etcetera)
23. Property (rings, keys, wallets, etcetera)

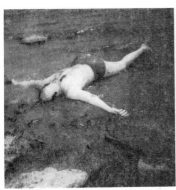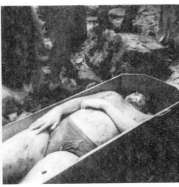

FIG. 18. Accidental drowning; subject twenty six years of age. Note loss of hair and general change in physical appearance after approximately one week in water—subject identified through dental work.

B. Specific procedure
 1. X-ray
 2. Special serological study of tissues
 3. Teeth (Fig. 18)
 4. Photography and fingerprinting
 5. Dental
 6. Other scientific procedures
III. Estimating approximate height in centimeters

Male

81.231 plus 1.880 times length of femur
70.714 plus 2.894 times length of humerus
78.807 plus 2.376 times length of tibia
86.465 plus 3.271 times length of radius

Female

73.163 plus 1.945 times length of femur
72.046 plus 2.754 times length of humerus
75.369 plus 2.352 times length of tibia
82.189 plus 3.343 times length of radius

(Pearson's Formula.)

—14—

BLOOD
SYNOPSIS

The collection and preservation of blood is one of the most important and consistent types of evidence in death investigation.

The collection, preservation and shipping of bloodstains and bloodstained objects is usually carried on by the investigator himself.

It is very important for the investigator, in all homicide investigations, to obtain, wherever possible, a sample of blood from the deceased and from the living suspect. It is further important that these blood samples be grouped and typed for future reference.

In addition to comparison purposes, bloodstains often tell many other stories, for example, through color and thickness the approximate time of death; through shape and size the direction from which it came, the distance that it fell and the part of the body from which it came (artery or vein).

If the investigating officer has any doubt as to his ability to collect and preserve the bloodstain and is unable to remove the object upon which it is contained, he should preserve it by placing some object over the stain itself, sealing same with adhesive or scotch tape, marking it so that the container cannot be removed without his knowledge, and preserving it in that condition until such time that an expert may be brought to the scene.
(Form 47—Benzidine Test for Blood)

BLOOD

I. General
  A. Is approximately 10% of total body weight
  B. The investigation of blood at the scene is very important as it may be an aid in approximating
    1. How long the victim actually lived after the death blow was inflicted
    Note: Dead bodies do not bleed except in drainage due to gravity
    2. What part of the body the blood came from
    3. Actual site of death blow
    4. Angle at which blow was struck
    5. Whether the body was moved
    6. Approximate time of death
    7. Possible identity of the accused
       AND/OR
       Of the deceased

II. Investigative points regarding blood
  A. Is it blood or not?
  B. If blood, is it human, animal, fish or fowl?
  C. If animal, what kind of animal?
  D. If human, to what group does it belong?
    1. Human blood separated into 4 major groups
       a. O—(approximately 45% of population)
       b. A—(approximately 40% of population)
       c. B—(approximately 10% of population)
       d. AB—(approximately 5% of population)

  2. Other blood groups, such as
   a. Rh System positive or negative
   b. M and N
   c. Multiple others
  Note: Very little likelihood of any one com-
    plete group occurring more than once
    in 2,500,000 people

 E. From what part of the body it comes
 F. Does it contain alcohol, carbon monoxide,
  etcetera?
 G. How old are the blood stains?
 H. Is it relative to the case under investigation?

III. Investigator's description of stains
 A. Shape
 B. Size
 C. Color (red, brown or black)
 D. Is the blood still moist, dry around the
  edges or entirely dry?
  THEN
 E. Stain sketched
 F. Photographed
  AND
 G. A sample taken

IV. Shape (Fig. 19)
 A. If in a spray, droplets will be found
 B. If shed in quantity, will seek lowest level
  and run in small streams
 C. If brisk, clothing will become saturated
 D. If clothing stained
  1. Small stains will not penetrate clothes
  SO
  2. Will show a bleeding from inside or
   outside

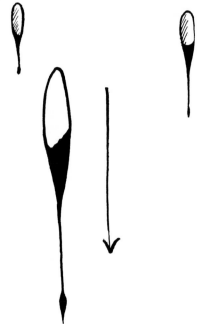

FIG. 19. Blood droplets, indicating direction of fall.

       3. Liquid blood will seep into small places (May be in wooden handle of knife or ax, even if blade itself is cleaned.)

V. Estimating age of blood
    A. A single drop of blood that falls on a dry surface such as a table or wood floor will dry completely in about one hour
    B. Where it is collected in pools, it may be several hours before it is dry, depending on the size and depth of the pool formed
    C. After a few hours, the blood usually is completely dry, making it very difficult to tell from the stains how long they have been there

BUT

D. In general, the older the blood stains the blacker they are

E. Aid to determining age of blood and amount of drying may be by running pencil through it to determine
    1. If still completely in liquid form
    2. If small thin line is created as blood goes together
    3. If blood becomes separated to approximately width of dividing pencil

VI. Estimating height of fall of blood (Fig. 20)

● A. Up to 20″—round and sharply delineated spots

★ B. 20″ to approximately 4½′—spots with prickly edges

✳ C. Over 4½′ — fine and close projections — needle-like splashes

\ D. Blood on wall can help tell direction of flow —exclamation mark pointed away from the bleeding

VII. Collection of evidence

A. General
    Whenever any doubt about removing, describe, diagram, photograph and cover, pending the arrival of the laboratory technician

B. Materials
    1. Scissors
    2. Clean glass container (test tube, bottle, etcetera)
    3. Distilled water
    4. Sterilized knife or razor
    5. Normal saline solution

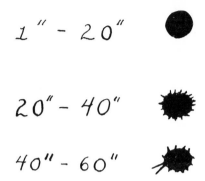

$1'' - 20''$

$20'' - 40''$

$40'' - 60''$

Fig. 20. Blood droplets, indicating height of fall.

      6. Adhesive tape
      7. Labels
  C. Fresh moist stains on clothing or the cloth
      1. Cut with clean scissors (not to exceed one-half of total stained area)
      2. Place in clean glass
      3. Cover specimen with normal saline solution
      4. Seal specimen in the container
      5. Allow remainder of stain to dry
      6. Pack when dry
      7. Pack in a clean box
      8. Protect stain areas
      9. For comparison, obtain blood of deceased, defendant or victim, adding anticoagulant
  D. Fresh, moist stains on solid objects or surfaces
      1. With clean instrument remove as much blood as possible
      2. Place blood in glass container or druggist fold

    3. Cover and seal
    4. Obtain comparison blood, as set forth above
    5. Allow remainder of blood to dry
    6. If possible, remove entire object upon which blood remains

E. Dry blood on solid object
    1. With clean knife, flake off particles of dry blood
    2. Place in clean glass container
    3. If possible, retain entire object upon which blood is located
    4. Obtain comparison samples as set forth above

F. Liquid blood for grouping
    1. Obtain at least 1 ounce from the victim
    2. Place in a sterile glass container
    3. Add anti-coagulant
    4. Obtain comparison blood

G. Other blood samples
    1. Liquid blood for drowning test
       All blood from left and right chambers of heart submitted in separate containers
    2. Liquid blood for carbon monoxide
       8 ounces of blood from the deceased
    3. Liquid blood for alcohol
       At least 3 ounces of blood of deceased

Note: In removing body, cover hands with bag to protect stains and prevent contamination thereof.

Note: In removing body, protect stains on clothing and other portions of body to prevent contamination and to prevent spread or distortion of stains.

Note: Use extreme care not to confuse other type
of stains (such as "coffee ground vomitus")
with blood stains. Oftentimes, vomitus resulting from a natural death may well re-
semble bloodstains, and thus confuse and
embarrass the investigator if premature conclusions are made (Fig. 21).

Note: Where anti-coagulant is unobtainable, liquid
blood should be immediately refrigerated.
(Fig. 22)

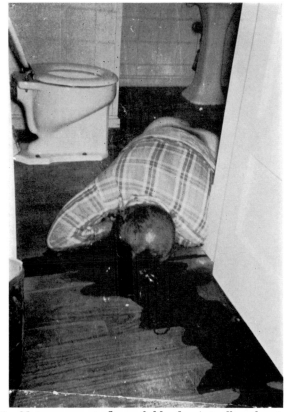

Fig. 21. Note apparent flow of blood. Actually, chemical test
showed large amount of blood-like substance was vomitus as
discolored by tobacco stain. Death natural.

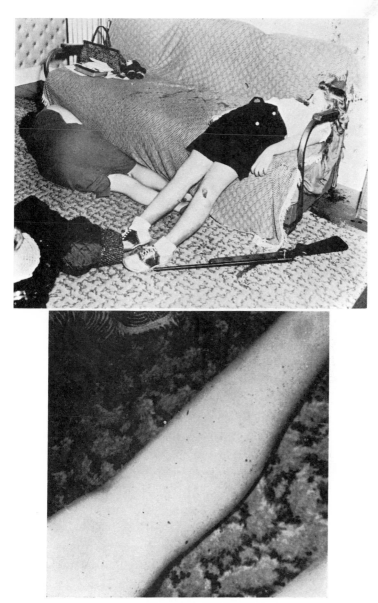

Fig. 22. Note droplets of blood on female body on the floor, indicating that the blood fell from a distance of less than 20″. Investigation indicated that the blood came from the hand of the younger female subject, demonstrating that the death of the woman preceded that of the child.

—15—

HAIR

I. Discovered as evidence under many different circumstances
    A. In grasp of a victim
    B. On his or her clothing
    C. On part of an automobile
    D. On a murder weapon, etcetera

II. Question
    A. Whether human or animal?
    B. Whether from living animal or from furs?
    C. Whether from the victim or the attacker?
    D. What is it doing where found?

III. Nomenclature (Fig. 23)
    A. Root
        1. Part normally embedded in skin
        2. May be round, oval, angular or hooked
    B. Tip
        1. Opposite end to root
        2. May be cut or may never have been cut
        3. May be split or crushed
    C. Shaft
        1. The section between root and tip
        2. Any part used to determine diameter
    D. Cuticle
        1. Scales covering hair on the outside
    E. Medulla
        1. Dark substance inside hair

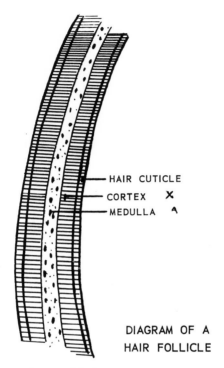

DIAGRAM OF A
HAIR FOLLICLE

Fig. 23. Nomenclature of hair.

F. Cortex
1. Between cuticle and medulla
2. Main bulk of hair
3. Contains coloring matter of hair
IV. Collection, preservation and shipping
A. Sample of hair, if obtained from victim, should be full hair, including the root
B. Hair should never be touched with finger (can contaminate with oil, water or dust)
C. Never allow to become lost or mixed with other hairs or fibers

D.   Angle cut hairs in shorter angles (coil them up if too long to fit in container otherwise)

E.   Place hair in round pill box or folded paper (druggist fold)

Note: Never place hair directly in an envelope (may become lost in creases)

F.   Hair on murder weapon
1.   Leave hair intact on weapon
2.   Label the weapon itself
3.   Draw a diagram showing position of hairs and their numbers
4.   Pack the weapon in such a manner that the hair cannot become lost

G.   Rape cases
1.   Pubic hairs of victim
2.   Any loose hairs in abdominal or thigh region

H.   By way of comparison, submit samples of hair from the victim, suspect or other possible sources of the unknown specimen

V.   General characteristics

A.   Clip hair
1.   Average diameter of less than .08 mm— male or female head hairs
2.   Average diameter of greater than .1 mm —beard

B.   Origin of hairs
1.   Angle of more than 3"—female head hairs
2.   Angle of 1½" to 3"
a.   Covered with grease—arm pits
b.   Curly and coarse
(1)   Male genitals, or
(2)   Female genitals

c. Wavy
    (1) Mustache
    (2) Scrotum
    (3) Genital orifice
3. Length of less than 1½″
  a. Brush-like
    (1) Torso, or
    (2) Legs, or
    (3) Arms
  b. Sharp tip
    (1) Eyelashes, or
    (2) Eyebrows and nostril

—16—

FINGERPRINTS
SYNOPSIS

Fingerprints are the only known type of identification of unknown persons that is absolutely infallible, provided that there is a record of those fingerprints which is accessible for comparison. Their pattern depends on the ridges which are present and of the papillary lines. Fingerprints are normally taken by rolling the fingers over an ink tab and then rolling them over a heavy piece of paper or cardboard to transfer the outlines of the papillary line to the cardboard. At times, it is not possible to roll the fingers on an ink tab or on the paper; however, it may be practicable to roll the ink pad on the finger and then to roll the paper on the finger. If the body is not rigid, there is very little problem in taking fingerprints from the corpse; however, when the body has become rigid it is impossible to literally roll the finger around the cardboard as there is a great danger of slipping and of the print itself being illegible; in the latter of these cases, it is suggested that the officer wait until such time that the pathologist can cut some tendons or muscles or loosen the fingers so that they may be rolled more easily.

Greater problems present themselves where the body is decomposed or has been burned.

It is possible at times to read the fingerprints directly from the fingers and classify them immediately, but this is not recommended except in cases of extreme emergency and for temporary purposes.

When the fingers have become shriveled up and dried, solution may be injected by needle underneath the skin to facilitate the taking of the prints.

Where the subject has been in water for some time, or on land in mud or dirt, the prints may be dirty and very unclear, and should be washed and/or dried; however, extreme care must be taken, in that some of the skin may be torn off during the process of washing and the print ruined. Prolonged period of time in water may also loosen the epidermis or top layer of the skin. In such a case the skin itself may be pulled or cut off and placed in a test tube filled with chemicals for cleaning and later examination. They should not be placed on paper or in an envelope, in that there is a great possibility of their drying up and sticking to the paper. Another method is removing the outer layer of skin, placing same over the expert's fingers and rolling these fingers on the pad of ink and on the cardboard. A fourth method is the removing of the skin, placing same between two glass plates and photographing.

It is recommended that no attempt to do any of these things be made by the officer on the scene, but that it be postponed until such time that it can be accomplished by experts and/or under their guidance (Fig. 24).

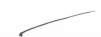

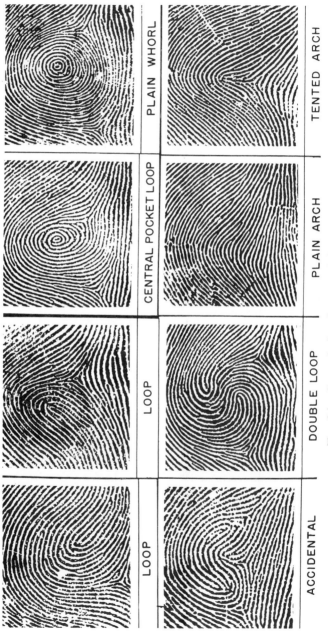

Fig. 24. General classification of fingerprints.

-17-

TEETH—DENTAL IDENTIFICATION

Dental identification procedures are a positive method for making identifications where the more routine methods cannot be used.

In the adult mouth there are normally 32 teeth, and the chances that any two individuals would have exactly the same teeth missing, the same teeth filled in the same area with the same filling material, and the missing teeth replaced by exactly the same type of prosthetic appliance are literally one in billions.

In making a dental identification, it is best to proceed with a definite formula in mind; a recommended procedure would be to chart the mouth in the following manner: starting with the upper right 3rd molar as tooth #1, proceed around the upper arch, giving each tooth a number, so that the upper left 3rd molar will be #16, and then dropping down to the lower left 3rd molar as #17 and then around to the lower right 3rd molar as #32.

This particular method is recommended because it is the one most widely used in dental charts of the dental departments of the Armed Forces, the Veterans Administration, and most public health agencies.

In making such a chart, the following must be carefully noted and recorded: (Fig. 25)

1) Missing teeth, i.e., #4, #12, etcetera
2) Filled teeth—and in what areas—and with what filling materials, i.e., #5— M O D —amalgam, #8 mesial silicate, #30 — do — gold inlay

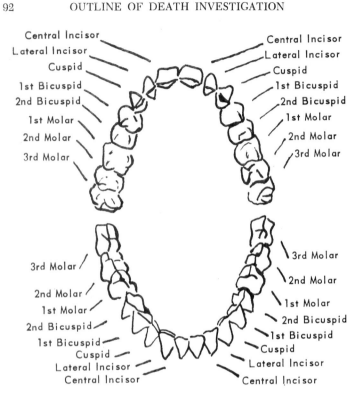

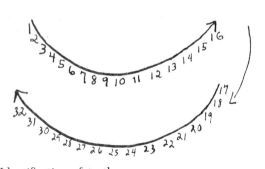

Fig. 25.　Identification of teeth.

Sometimes decayed teeth may also aid in identification, so it is wise to chart these areas too.

   3) Replaced teeth, i.e.
      (a) Fixed bridge; #3 to #6 with ¾ crown on #6 and no inlay on #3
      (b) i.e., lower partial denture replacing lower 4 anteriors
   4) Other characteristics
      (a) Devitalized teeth
      (b) Deciduous teeth
      (c) Supernumerary teeth
      (d) Unusual spaces between the teeth
      (e) Unusual anatomy and structure of the individual teeth, i.e., peg shaped laterals, rotated bicuspids, fissures on the central or lateral incisor resulting from chemical staining—fluorides, etc.

At times it may be necessary to make casts of the mouth in order to make more positive identifications. This, of

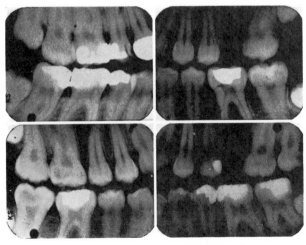

Fig. 26. X-Ray bite wing examination technique.

course, is the only means for a dental identification in an edentulous mouth; the cast should be carefully examined for unusual bony formations.

It is recommended that x-rays of teeth be taken for purpose of permanent record, and to establish identifying characteristics that may not be apparent to the examining eye. (Fig. 26).

(Forms 21 and 22—Dental Charts.)

TEETH

I. General
   A. Most durable of all animal tissue
   B. Can be used by investigator to establish
       1. Identity
       2. Age
       3. Race
       4. Sex
       5. Characteristics
II. Development
   A. Six months
       First teeth starting with incisors (milk teeth)
   B. Twelve months
       First temporary molars
   C. Eighteen months
       Canines
   D. Two years
       Second temporary molars
   E. Between two to six years
       Temporary teeth complete
   F. Six years
       First permanent molars
   G. Six to twelve years
       Temporary teeth replaced by permanent ones
   H. Twelve years
       Second permanent molars
   I. Eighteen to twenty-two years
       1. Wisdom teeth erupt
       2. Thirty-two teeth altogether

III. Examination
    A.   Dentist should be used
    B.   Record on dental chart
    C.   Take x-rays
        1. For defects
        2. For structure
        3. For fillings
           a. Place
           b. Type
           c. Characteristics
    D.   Dentures
        1. Type
        2. Number of teeth
        3. Structure
        4. Material
        5. Manufacturer
        6. Other identifying marks

—18—

POST-MORTEM CHANGES
SYNOPSIS

In the investigation of homicide cases, where the death itself was not personally witnessed, it is necessary to make a determination as to the time of death. This is important in the establishment of a corpus delicti, the placing of the accused at the scene at a given time, and either corroborating or disproving his alibis.

The establishment of time of death is also important in civil matters. By example, it could be necessary to establish which one of any given number of people expired first, for the purpose of inheritance; in Workmen's Compensation Cases, it could become necessary to determine whether the death occurred within the scope of the deceased's employment; and where there are insurance policies, time of death could play an important part if the question arises whether the policy was in force at the time of death, or whether payment could be restricted because of a policy limitation (for example, a one year suicide clause).

In approximating the time of death, physical clues in or about the scene can be of greater help to the investigator than an autopsy or medical examination by a physician either on the scene or at the morgue. Most common clues are a broken watch, dated newspapers, milk or mail, presence of food on the table (particularly where an autopsy will indicate that the subject ate this food and the progress of its digestion), electric lights being on or off, the subject's manner of dress, presence of foliage, dirt or mud in the house or on the subject, determination of when the subject was last seen, heard from or talked to (Fig. 27).

Examination of clues often requires additional help which can come from neighboring universities, institu-

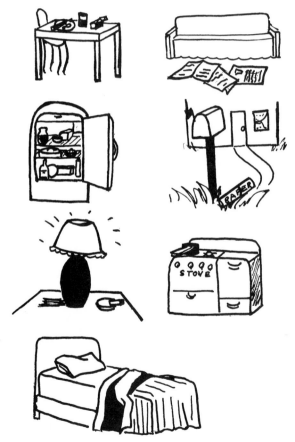

Fig. 27. Household clues determining time of death.

tions and factories that might employ expert personnel. To utilize this help, the investigator must do three things: firstly, he should familiarize himself with the expert personnel that is available in his community; secondly, he should be ever vigilant of the minute clue that these experts might use; and, thirdly, he should protect and safeguard this all-important bit of evidence, so as not to contaminate or distort it before examination by these experts.

Insects and bacteria that have found a home, reproduced and grown on and in certain portions of the victim's body (particularly in the apertures such as his nostrils, mouth, eyes and ears), earth and foliage beneath the subject or within his clothes, and other such clues which are beyond the comprehension of the average investigator, can well give the qualified specialist and scientist important clues as to both time of death and approximate location where the injury causing the death was inflicted.

It must be emphasized that an all-important bridge is destroyed—a bridge that cannot again be crossed—when the body is moved. Time often may be an essence in the reaching of a scene, but, once that scene is reached, secured and protected, time is no longer a factor in the investigation of the clues therein. The investigator should have no reluctance, when any doubt exists as to the importance of a clue which is beyond his ability to comprehend, secure or analyze, to call upon such experts as pathologists, medical technologists, botanists, zoologists, or the like, to study, remove and interpret them, and thus help in establishing a time of death and in the reconstructing of the death scene.

As important as the investigation itself is the realization on the part of the investigator that a premature and inaccurate release of what he thinks is an APPROXIMATE time of death can and probably will be the best alibi that an accused can use to win his freedom. Thusly, in spite of constant interrogation and pressure, the investigator should not release to either the news media or any other person a premature estimation of time of death. He should rather wait until all the clues are carefully examined, witnesses interrogated and consultations between the investigator and the medic held, before releasing his "estimated and approximate" (and not "exact") time of death.

The inability to state an exact time of death is not an indication of ignorance; rather it is honesty and common sense that is bound to pay off at a subsequent trial.

POST-MORTEM CHANGES

I. Immediate signs of death
  A. Cessation of breathing
  B. Cessation of pulse
  C. Loss of muscle tone in eyeballs
  D. Changes in pupil
  Note: Oftentimes it is difficult for the layman to determine whether a subject is alive or dead; if any question exists, then the subject should be presumed to be alive and the officer should act accordingly until a qualified medical practitioner actually pronounces him dead.
II. Early post-mortem changes
  A. Goose skin—cool places, occurring
    1. Soon after death, and
    2. Lasting up to 24 hours
  B. Loss of body heat (approximately 98.6° F. during life)
    1. Certain modes of dying may cause a terminal rise (increase in temperature)
    2. Rate of cooling
      a. Depends on difference between the temperature of the body and its environment
      AND
      b. Upon surface area of the body exposed for each unit of heat it contains
      AND
      c. On type of surface upon which body is lying

AND

d. On amount of clothing subject may be wearing

  Note: Rate slows as temperature of body approaches that of environment

  Note: Heat is lost from the body by conduction, convection and radiation

  Note: Damp or wet body will cool more rapidly owing to evaporation of the moisture

  Note: Covering or clothing will delay cooling

3. Cooling

a. When the room temperature is 72° F., and the body temperature has been reduced to 72° F., then it may be assumed that the person has been dead 24 to 36 hours

b. The body loses approximately 2½° temperature the first hour, approximately 1½° temperature for the next 18 hours, and approximately 1° temperature thereafter, until the body reaches the temperature of its environment

4. Recording

a. Rectally or in the liver

Note: When there is an indication of murder or sodomy and the rectum might be a factor, then that rectum must be undisturbed

    b. Recording of the temperature of the environment or the room in which the body is found

    c. At least 2 recordings of the temperature of both the body and the environment should be taken—the said recordings being made in 2 to 3 hour intervals

III. Rigor mortis

 A. General

  Post-mortem contraction of the voluntary and involuntary muscle fibers due to breakdown of enzymes of substances in the muscles

 B. Factors affecting

  1. Warm environment and cold environment

   a. Chilled body—rigor more rapid in onset and slower in leaving

   b. Warm body—reverse process in "a"

  2. Physical activity at time of death

   a. Certain types of exertion, nervous tension and manners of death may speed rigor mortis

   b. Physical make-up of subject may either hasten or delay rigor mortis

 C. Time

  1. Commences 2 to 4 hours

   a. First in eyelids and face

   b. Then in neck, arms, trunk and legs

  2. Full development 12 to 18 hours

  3. Persists 12 to 18 hours

  4. Disappears in same order

D. Notes
   1. Once rigor is fully developed, then broken, it will not reappear
   2. Rigor mortis in and of itself is a very unreliable test to determine time of death
   3. Embalming—creates chemical stiffening (Fig. 28)

IV. Cadaveric spasm (Fig. 29.)
   A. General
      1. Immediate stiffening of a particular

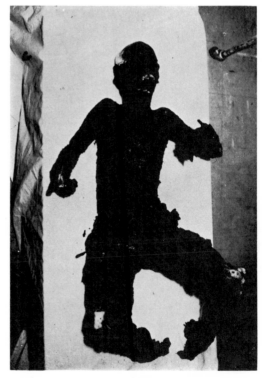

FIG. 28. Note pugilistic attitude of subject. Rigor mortis created by burning.

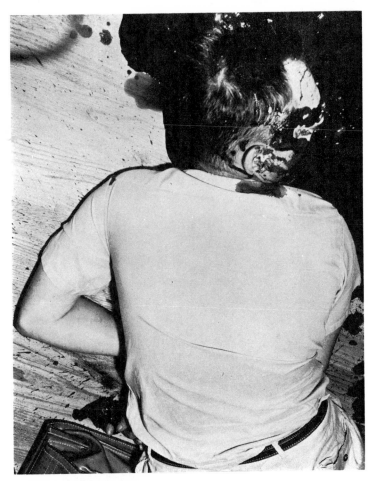

FIG. 29. Cadaveric spasm.

       group of muscles, confined to a *single*
       group of muscles, e.g., hands or arms
2. Cause unknown
3. Death must be
   a. Sudden

   b. While subject is in a state of nervous
      tension
   c. Muscle groups must be in a state of
      physical activity at time of death
B.   Time
   1. Immediately after death
   2. Does *not* pass off after time—remains
      until after putrefaction
Note: Cadaveric spasm cannot be imitated by
      another person
V. Lividity (Fig. 30)
   A.   General
      1. Caused by settling of blood through
         gravity and a dilation of blood vessels
      2. Purplish discoloration of part of body
         nearest surface upon which subject is
         lying

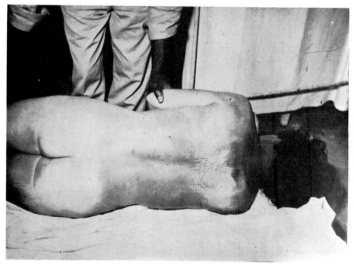

Fig. 30. Lividity.

B. Important
1. In determining time of death
AND
2. Obtaining knowledge as to whether the body was moved after death
Note: Lividity will not occur where pressure is created on a body by the surface upon which it is lying,
OR
May not appear where the person has lost a great deal of blood before expiring
C. Testing
1. When it first develops lividity will disappear when pressure is applied by finger, and skin will become white on touch; then when pressure is released, the lividity will reappear
2. After 4 to 5 hours, the blood becomes clotted and will not disappear on pressure or by moving
D. Time
1. Process starts immediately at death, with the cessation of circulation of the blood
2. First seen ½ to 4 hours after death
3. Full intensity 12 hours after death
E. Notes
1. Person with circulatory failure—lividity is seen shortly after death
2. Sudden death—first seen in a series of blotches over dependent parts
3. Will not shift with moving of body
4. Disappears after putrefaction has decomposed blood

       5. Importance—distribution and color

F.   *NOT* to be confused with bruises

    1. Standard indications of lividity as compared to bruises (see sub-paragraph 2)

       a. Affected by gravity — discoloration always in portion of body closest to surface

       b. Discoloration uniform throughout body area affected

       c. Discoloration contains no abrasions

       d. Discoloration contains no elevation of skin

    2. Standard indications of bruises as compared to lividity (see sub-paragraph 1)

       a. Not affected by gravity

       b. Portions discolored not uniform in coloring

       c. Examination of discolored areas either by eye or microscope will show some type of abrasion

       d. Usually accompanied by elevation of skin in bruised area

    3. A third type of discoloration is post-mortem discoloration, which can be confused with lividity and bruising

Note: Where in doubt as to whether discoloration is lividity, bruising or post-mortem discoloration, autopsy should be performed, and determination and classification should be made by microscopic examination

Note: A person's blood comprises 10% of his total weight.

VI. Putrefaction (Fig. 31)
  A. General
    1. Destruction of soft tissues by bacteria and enzymes or ferments
    2. Accompanied by evolution of gas
  B. Time
    1. In temperature above 70° F., putrefaction will be hastened
    2. In summertime can occur within 24 hours
    3. In wintertime may take as long as 10 or 14 days
  C. Signs
    1. First, greenish discoloration of abdomen and genitals

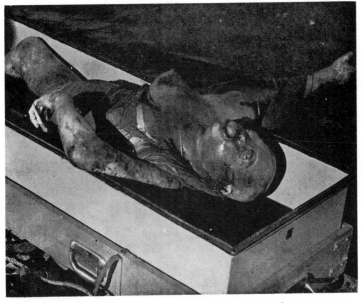

Fig. 31. Death by drowning. In water five days during summer season.

    2. Veins in skin—blue or purplish (due to pigments of decomposing blood—called marbling)

    3. After 5 to 7 days thin-walled vesicles appear—may rupture, emitting foul-smelling fluid

    4. After rupture dries—yellow parchment-like membrane

    5. About 7 days

       a. Abdomen swells—body bloats (from accumulation of gas)

       b. Fluid emits from mouth and nose, the source of this fluid being the lungs and stomach

       c. Rectum may empty

    6. May continue until all tissues disappear and skeleton alone remains (Fig. 32)

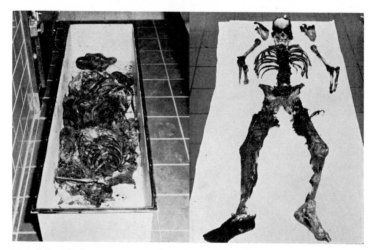

FIG. 32. Skeleton remains found in field during summer season. Subject dead approximately thirty days. Probable partial devourment by animals.

Note: Inaccurate in determining time of death

Note: When bloating and darkening occurs, it may be difficult to determine the race and color of the deceased

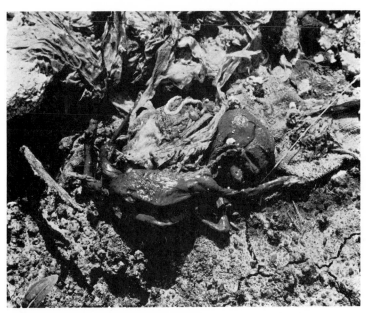

FIG. 33. Mummification of fetus.

VII. Mummification (Fig. 33)
    A. General
        Dehydration of body tissues (loss of liquids)
    B. Requires a hot dry temperature (deserts)
    C. Time
        1. It may take as long as a year for mummification to set in
        2. It may last for many years

Note: Mummification may set in in any type of
temperature or climate in a new-born
baby, in that such a baby is sterile and
has no bacteria to cause putrefaction or
decay from within

VIII. Adipocere formation
    A. General
        Hydrogenation of body fats into fatty acids
    B. Identification
        1. Sweetish smell
        2. Yellowish-white, soap-like substance
        3. Most prevalent where fat deposits
           (cheeks, abdominal wall, buttocks, etc.)
        4. Mostly in warm, damp conditions
        5. Where present internal organs usually
           in good shape (dehydrated and mumi-
           fied in process)
    C. Time
        Within few weeks in summertime

IX. Water
    A. Swelling of epidermis of skin of finger tips
        —starts few hours after death
    B. Hands swollen after several days
    C. Outer layer of skin—separated from inner
        layer within 5 to 6 days
    D. Skin and nails separate from body within 2
        to 3 weeks
    E. Seaweed vegetation within 8 to 10 days
    F. Floating
        1. Warm water 8 to 10 days, (Fig. 34).
        2. Cool water 2 to 3 weeks

X. Eye changes
    A. Pupil dilates—begins to restrict and become
        small—5 to 7 hours

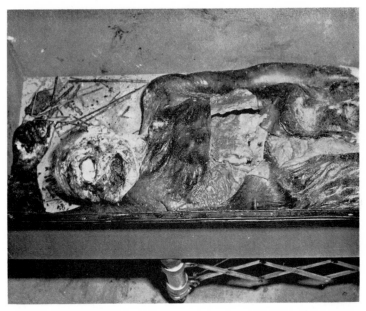

Fɪɢ. 34. Advanced putrefaction. In warm water eight to ten days.

B. Pupil regains position of equilibrium—18 to 20 hours

C. Cornea becomes cloudy—12 to 20 hours

XI. Chemical tests (spinal fluid, gastric contents, eye changes, etc.)

XII. Post-mortem attacks—animals, insects, etc. (Fig. 35)

XIII. Plants under and near body

Note: Samples should be taken of plant growth under the body and plant growth of the area surrounding the body to be later examined by a qualified person

Note: Vegetation generally will lose its green coloration (chlorophyll) in approximately 5

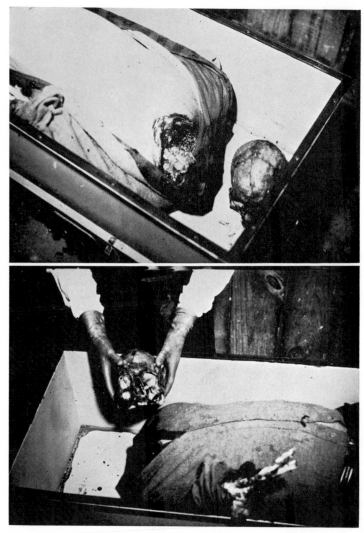

FIG. 35. Subject found in his own home. Partially devoured.
Four dogs locked in house.

to 7 days because of loss of sun and other
light

XIV.   Foliage and insects (Fig. 36)

Molds, foliage and insects may grow and repro-
duce upon and within the body.   Eggs and lar-

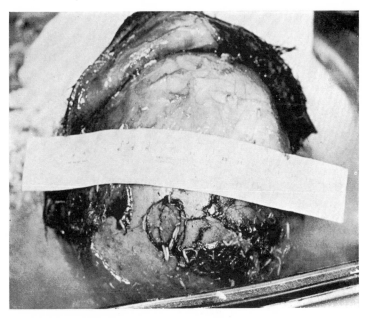

FIG. 36.   Maggot infestation.

vae might be laid, usually in the lips and nostrils.
These should be protected and preserved, to be
examined by those specialized in the particular
field as another aid in determining time of death

XV.   Stomach contents

A.   Stomach full and digestion not extensive
(death shortly after meal)

   B.   Stomach empty (death occurred 4 to 6 hours after meal)
   C.   Small intestine also empty (death occurred 12 hours or more after meal)
XVI.   Associated events to determine time and date of death
   A.   Examples
        1. Electric lights on or off
        2. Newspapers (dates)
        3. Mail (when delivered)
        4. Meals (whether on table, on stove or in refrigerator)
        5. Watch or clock
   Note: Hair and nails do *not* grow after death
   Note: Embalming handicaps investigation
   Note: Both an examination of the body and investigation of the circumstances surrounding the death are important and essential in aiding the investigator to determine the approximate time of death

—19—

UNEXPECTED "NATURAL" DEATHS

SYNOPSIS

Every sudden or unexpected death presents a problem to the physician who pronounces the subject dead and to the investigator and coroner who is notified thereof.

Unless the physician has some personal knowledge of and familiarity with the person and circumstances, has recently treated the subject, and can accurately diagnose the cause of death, he should not hazard a guess but should simply report same to the coroner as death from unknown natural causes.

When the patient dies after having been ill for some time and having been under physician's care during this illness, the death is not considered unexpected or unknown, and hospital, physician and clinical history can provide satisfactory explanation of the demise. When these factors or any of them are not present, the death is considered unexpected, unexplained, and, as such, coroner's cases.

Actually, the number of such unexplained and unknown (although the death may later be determined to be from natural causes), deaths that come to the attention of the coroner's office comprises more than fifty per cent of all cases handled by that office.

Of the sudden deaths:

(1) Heart disease takes the greatest toll, the more specific causes being acute coronary thrombosis, acute coronary insufficiency, cardiac failure in arteriosclerotic heart

disease and aorta (rupture of the aneurysm). If the adult is apparently in perfect health and suddenly falls dead, chances are that he died of a coronary disease.

(2) Brain—cerebral hemorrhage is usually due to hypertension ("stroke").

(3) Lungs—pulmonary embolism is not usually the cause of a sudden death and sometimes occurs if the patient has been bedridden for a long time or has not used some extremity. Other common lung diseases causing sudden death are acute pneumonia ("Asian Flu") and aspiration of vomitus. There is usually a cause for this aspiration.

(4) Liver—acute liver insufficiency—cirrhosis (sometimes caused by excessive drinking over a long period of time).

(5) Women in childbearing age come to death often as a result of air embolism following an abortion or massive hemorrhage following an abortion or delivery.

(6) Sudden death in the "crib" in infancy. Contrary to popular belief comparatively very few children actually come to their deaths as a result of suffocation, but rather from natural causes. One cause is interstitial pneumonia, which is frequent in infants up to 9 months of age, and is usually seen in the fall, winter or early spring. It strikes without warning or previous symptoms and kills the child quickly, because of the child's lack of immunity. Many children also die from aspiration of stomach contents, associated with pneumonia or whooping cough. Actually, cases of accidental strangulation are usually confined to venetian blind cords, plastic sleeping bags, etcetera. Congenital diseases also account for a large number of infant deaths. In the case of infants, more than in adults, death unexpectedly coming from natural causes brings with it a

feeling of guilt and recrimination, as well as uncertainty as to the health of other members of the family. Autopsies to determine the exact cause are necessary for the protection of all concerned, society and the family, and for the peace of mind and conscience of the immediate family (Fig. 37).

The officer or coroner does not justify anyone by allowing a doubtful case to "slip by" as a natural death. He may unknowingly be protecting a murderer, hiding a suicide or depriving the family of compensation or double indemnity (accidental death).

No unattended death is natural per se. Only after the suspicion of the investigator is allayed and after examination of the body shows the absence of evidence of trauma can the death be determined a natural one.

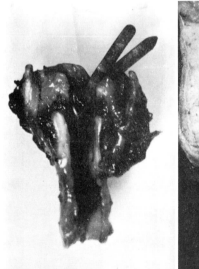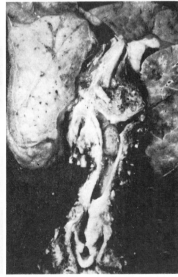

FIG. 37. Deaths by "apparent" natural causes. Actual cause of death in one case was swallowing of a bean and in the other swallowing of a paper clip.

On the other hand, the fact that the victim has come to his death under circumstances which might indicate violence should not be construed as a violent death by the officer until such time that it is reported to the coroner's office, and by means of either an autopsy or other type post-mortem examination or by consulting with the victim's family and physician, if any, it is discovered that this person did, in effect, die from an existing sickness or an acute attack of some sort. A surprisingly large percentage of suspicious deaths involving injuries to the deceased, a great amount of loss of blood, wrecked vehicles (especially where a stationary object has been struck by the said vehicle) and "drownings," are, after careful investigation and medical examination, found to be natural deaths, and that the violence actually resulted after the subject has, in effect, deceased. The most common causes of this type of very sudden deaths are coronary ailments.

Finally, statistical death averages which are compiled by such agencies as safety councils, highway departments, coroner's offices, etcetera, can be and are falsely and erroneously computed when causes of death are not accurately reported. The most flagrant example of this error are many of the so-called "automobile fatalities," which, in effect, are natural deaths wherein the victim had first suffered an attack, which attack caused not only the accident but the death itself.

(Form 27—Apparent Natural Death Report)

—20—

DOCTORS AND SUDDEN "NATURAL" DEATHS

I. Necessary for a doctor to pronounce subject dead in *all* cases
    A. Even where death is "obvious"
    B. *Not* officially dead until so pronounced by doctor

II. Doctor
    A. SHOULD
        1. Inquire of police and other persons as to circumstances
        2. Examine deceased and clothing
            a. Notice and note arrangement of clothing
            b. Examine body externally for signs of injury
        3. Inquire and determine whether body was moved before his arrival
        4. Make notes on position of body, etc.
        5. Record temperature, lividity, rigor, etc.
        6. Note medications, etc.
        7. Superintend removal of body
        8. Immediately notify coroner and/or police where a natural cause of death is not certain and/or he is not able to sign the death certificate
    B. SHOULD NOT
        1. Sign certificate unless he has treated deceased

2. Interfere with police investigation
3. Touch anything, especially weapons
4. Leave before police arrive
5. Smoke or throw cigarette ashes, matches, etc., on scene
6. Conject on cause of death

III. Investigator
   A. SHOULD
      1. Eliminate all questions of suspicion
      2. Determine all the circumstances concerned
      3. Acquaint himself with all members of the household

   Note: Failure of any member of the household to cooperate might lead to conclusion that all is not well

      4. Determine exertions or complaints
      5. Obtain history of past injuries, even minor ones, which could have contributed to the death
      6. Look at the body
      7. Check the area and the body for
         a. Signs of struggle
         b. Signs of poisons
         c. Signs of medications
         d. Signs of anything else suspicious
      8. If any doubt appears
         a. Notify the coroner
         b. Summon police homicide division

   B. SHOULD NOT
      1. Form conclusions of his own
         BUT
         Wait until a more detailed examination and investigation is completed

   2. Release any false or misleading information which might be embarrassing to the officer or the family

   3. Allow the moving or destroying of anything which could later aid in the determination of the exact cause of death

Note: No unattended death is natural per se

—21—

ABORTION

I. General
    A. Definition (Fig. 38)
       Emptying of uterus prematurely (emptying of uterus before 28 weeks of gestation is called miscarriage)
    B. Types
       1. Natural, caused by
          a. Defect in, ovum or its membranes
          b. Some disease of the mother
       2. Accidental
          a. Blow, shock or other trauma
            (Rare unless injury to mother is severe)
       3. Therapeutic
          a. Interruption of pregnancy to conserve the health or save the life of the mother
       4. Criminal
          a. Interruption of pregnancy without valid medical means
            OR
          b. Induced without valid medical reasons

II. Persons involved in abortion
    A. Patient (usually dead)
    B. Husband or other member of family
    C. Illicit lover
    D. Abortionist

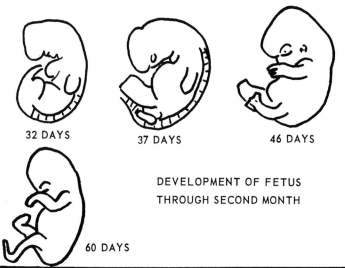

32 DAYS   37 DAYS   46 DAYS

DEVELOPMENT OF FETUS
THROUGH SECOND MONTH

60 DAYS

DEVELOPMENT OF FETUS IN FEMALE

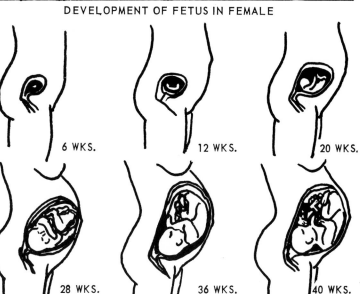

6 WKS.   12 WKS.   20 WKS.

28 WKS.   36 WKS.   40 WKS.

Fig. 38. Development of human embryo.

III. Methods
    A. First period (end of first month)
        1. Violent exercises
        2. Hot baths
        3. Violence to the abdominal region to promote congestion of blood
        4. Purgatives (castor oil or the like)
        5. Douches
        6. Drugs and chemicals
        7. Electric shocks to stimulate the womb
    B. Second period (end of second month)
        1. Drugs
           a. Will not work unless the quantity is so great that it actually endangers life
           b. By mouth
              (1) To make muscles and uterus contract and squeeze out pregnancy
              (2) Violent purgatives to increase menstrual flow
              (3) Hormone preparations
              (4) Metals
           c. Injected instruments
              (1) Inject fluid to strip the fetal sac and placenta
              (2) Syringe containing a carbolic soap
           d. Penetration
           e. Foreign bodies inserted—for example
              (1) Catheters
              (2) Darning needles
              (3) Wires
              (4) Pencils
    C. Third period (third or fourth month)
        1. To puncture pregnancy

2. To detach fetus
3. Instruments
   a. Pastes
      (1) Soapy paste
      (2) Creosol
      (3) Lye
   b. Soapy water (air)
   c. Instruments

IV. Results
   A. Once fetus is killed or destroyed, body will naturally eject same
   B. While mother alive
      1. Convulsions
      2. Critically ill
      3. Diarrhea
      4. Bleeding
   C. Rapid death
      1. Vagal shock
      2. Hemorrhage
      3. Embolism (air finding way into blood stream)
   D. Delayed deaths
      1. Renal infections
      2. Other infections
      3. Damage to organs
      4. Poisoning
      5. Shock
      6. Loss of blood
      7. Embolism
   Note: Delayed deaths usually two or more days after abortion

V. Investigation
   A. Unexpected deaths in healthy women of childbearing age

B. Bleeding from vagina
C. Deaths in unusual places, such as hotel rooms, dormitories, etc.
D. High fever or chills
E. Stupor
F. Pale or anemic cases
G. Evidence
  1. Drugs
  2. Paste or drugs
  3. Instruments
  4. Douche bags
  5. Clothing disarrangement
  6. Bloody gauze or clothing
  7. Spots on floor or bed
  8. Bloody wires, coat holders, etc.
  9. Atomizers
H. Place to search
  1. Patient's home
  2. Abortionist's office
  3. Hotel room or the like
VI. Elements of proof
  A. Pregnancy
  B. Duration of pregnancy
  C. Evidence of criminal abortion
  D. Method of procuring the abortion
  E. Relationship between the time of abortion and time of death
  F. Relation between the abortion and death
  G. Intent to cause an abortion
VII. Dying declarations
  A. In case of abortion, dying declarations are very essential
  B. Important elements
    1. That victim was pregnant

    2. Agreement between victim and abortion-
        ist to terminate pregnancy

C. Witnesses to the agreement

D. The abortion itself
    1. When
    2. Where
    3. How

E. Circumstances occurring to victim after the
    abortion

F. Definite identification of the abortionist

—22—

ANOXIA

I. Definition
   Failure of oxygen to reach the cells of the body

II. Types
   A. Anoxic
      Oxygen cannot gain access to blood stream—(high altitudes, asphyxia, drowning, lung disease, nitrous oxide)
   B. Stagnant
      Failure of circulation
      (Shock, cardiac failure)
   C. Histotoxic
      Cell unable to utilize oxygen which is available from blood stream—(hypnotics, barbiturates, cyanide, carbon dioxide)
   D. Anemic
      Blood unable to carry enough oxygen — (carbon monoxide)

—23—

ASPHYXIA

I. Definition
- A. Results when respiratory interchange between air in lung alveoli and blood in pulmonary capillaries is interrupted. Red blood cells cannot replenish oxygen supply and carbon dioxide cannot be discharged from blood into lung
    1. Obstruction of passage of air to the lungs
    2. Prevention of diffusion of oxygen across pulmonary membrane
    3. Difficulties encountered in blood-carrying mechanism (carbon monoxide, pulmonary embolism)
    4. Cellular inability to use oxygen (i.e., cyanide poisoning)
- B. Symptoms
    1. Lividity more than normal
    2. Cyanosed
       (Because asphyxia due to mechanical interference with respiration, leading to fatal oxygen lack)
    3. Bladder and lower bowels may empty
    4. Vomiting may occur
       (Because manner of interference with respiratory permits)
    5. Petechial hemorrhages on skin, especially eyelids (also common in narcotic poisoning)

6. Vagal shock
    To vagus nerves—can cause cessation of
    heart due to reflex impulse
7. Heart may be dilated
8. Lung may be heavy
9. Bronchial tree has some material

Note: Can be natural or traumatic

II. Strangulation
    A. Definition
        1. Asphyxia when neck is constricted or
           compressed
        2. The weight of the body *not* contributing
           to the compression
           BY
           a. Manual
           b. Ligature
      Note: Usually homicide
    B. Mechanism and cause of death
        1. Mechanical asphyxia
        2. With or without vagal shock
    C. Examination of body
        1. Petechial hemorrhage in eyes, face or
           neck
        2. Blood-tinged fluid from mouth and nose
        3. Tip of tongue between teeth and some-
           times swollen
        4. Face congested and cyanosed
        5. Assailant's marks
           a. Abrasions from struggle and finger-
              nails
           b. Bruises from struggle and pressure of
              fingers
           c. Bruises from fall

      6. Ligature
         a. Lower on neck—(at "Adam's Apple")
         b. Straight across neck
         c. Equal marks around neck
      7. Victim should be examined for
         a. Signs of struggle
         b. Fingernails—skin of assailant
         c. Hair or clothing clenched in hand
      8. Scene

III. Hanging (Fig. 39)
    A. Definition
       1. Caused by compression of neck by a ligature—caused by
         a. Weight of suspended or partially suspended body
         b. Consciousness
            (1) Rapid loss with
            (2) Movement of unconscious convulsion—caused by cerebral anoxia
    B. Ligature
       1. Knot
         a. Usually on left or right side rather than in front or back
           AND
         b. Usually rises behind ear to point of suspension
       2. Level
         a. Knot at higher level than remainder of ligature—due to act of suspension
         b. Main force opposite point of suspension
       Note: In removal of ligature, preserve ligature and knot intact (Fig. 40)

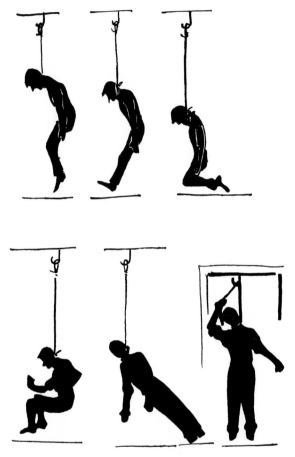

Fig. 39. Showing positions of suicidal hanging.

    3. Impression around neck
        a. Most prominent on part opposite knot
        b. Abrasion—parchment-like yellow
        c. Mark depends on
            (1) Composition of ligature
            (2) Texture of pattern reproduced on skin

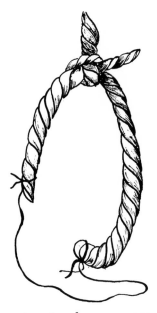

Fig. 40. Correct way to cut and remove rope.

       (3) Width and multiplicity of ligature will influence depth of impression

       (4) Weight of body suspended

       (5) Degree of suspension

       (6) Length of time suspended (longer suspended —deeper groove)

   d. Tightness of encircling ligature depends on

       (1) Free running of the noose

       (2) Length of ligature

       (3) Weight of body

   e. Ligature tends to slip upwards on neck toward the face—stopped by jaws

   C.   Cause of death
1. Ligature presses
2. Constricts respiratory passages, arteries, veins and their endings
3. Tongue may be forced backward, mechanically blocking the airway
4. Pressure of less than 8 pounds sufficient to cause cerebral anoxia and unconsciousness
5. Pull of 36½ pounds—necessary to occlude vertebral arteries
6. Between 8 pounds and 36 pounds—sufficient to occlude trachea

   Note: Ligature need *not* encircle entire neck

7. Mode of death influenced by
   a. Obstruction to airway
   b. Obstruction to blood circulation to head
      (1) Venous return
      (2) Arterial supply
   c. Sudden rise in venous and capillary pressure due to upward pull and compression

   D.   General appearances (Fig. 41)
1. Petechial hemorrhages (eyes and near ligature)
2. Congestion of head and neck (above ligature)
3. Protrusion and swelling of tongue
4. Injuries by anoxia, convulsive movements
5. Lividity (head and face remain congested)

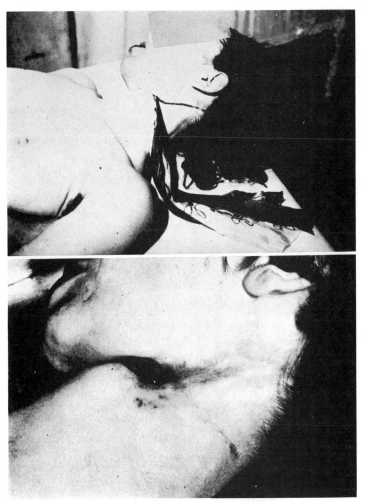

FIG. 41. Suicide by hanging—ligature and ligature mark.

E. Accidental hanging (3 groups)
  1. Experiments in self-suspension
  2. While at work or play
  3. Sex deviation (Fig. 42)

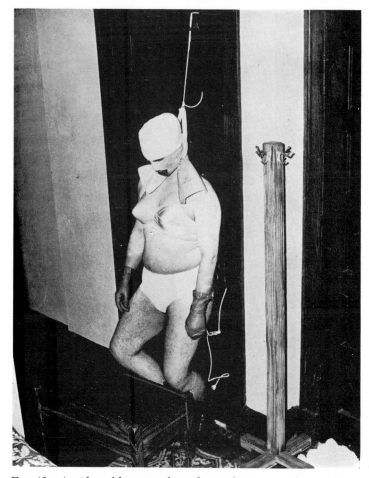

Fɪɢ. 42.   Accidental hanging through misadventure and masochism.
Subject is a male.

     a. Anoxia enhances sexual stimulation
     b. Rapid loss of consciousness—important
        tant
     c. Scene

        (1) Evidence of abnormal sexual behavior
        (2) Evidence of past practices
        (3) Evidence of attempt to leave no visible marks
            (cloth below ligature)
        (4) No evidence of suicidal intent
        (5) Masochism
        (6) Pornography
        (7) Transvestism (dressed in woman's clothing)
        (8) Mirrors
        (9) Semen—ejaculation

Note: Mark produced by ligature can be reproduced after death, if body is suspended within 2 hours of death

F. Investigation
    1. Do *not* untie or destroy knots
    2. Search area for
        a. Signs of struggle
        b. Suicide notes
        c. Rest of ligature or place from which ligature was taken
        d. Indications of prior attempts
        e. Other clues
        f. What subject was doing—for possibility of accident
        g. Stepping-off point

G. Background of victim for
    1. Prior suicide attempts
    2. Possible despondency
    3. Health
    4. Financial conditions
    5. Threats of suicide

      6. Recent behavior

      7. Other possible motives

  H. Search then for

      1. Struggle

      2. Notes—identify handwriting

      3. Signs of sex perversion

  I. Examine subject for

      1. Pressure marks or nails on neck, and bruises

      2. Dirt or leaves on subject

      3. Ground beneath the subject

      4. Blood or saliva flowing in wrong direction

      5. Fingernails of subject for possible struggle

      6. Lividity marks

      7. Rigor mortis

      8. Urine or excretion under body

      9. Where and how rope was tied

     10. Knots used

     11. Angle of bruise

  J. Determination of difference between strangulation by ligature and hanging

      1. Scene—hanging

         a. Suicide note

         b. No struggle

         c. No other injuries

      2. Scene—strangulation

         a. Other injuries besides the ligature marks

         b. Signs of struggle

      3. Ligature—hanging

         a. In position on body comparable with mark beneath it

        b. Ligature at the "Adam's apple" or above (upper thyroid level)
        c. Rises to point of suspension (highest point being at the knot)
        d. Neck most deeply grooved at point opposite that of suspension
    4. Ligature—strangulation
        a. Ligature may not be with the body
        b. Ligature below the "Adam's apple" horizontally
        c. Neck encircled horizontally
        d. Ligature marks evenly grooved completely around the neck

IV. Smothering
  A. Definition
    Asphyxia by obstruction to external airway, nose and mouth
  B. External appearances
    1. Cyanosed
    2. Petechial hemorrhages
    3. Blood-tinged froth or mucous from mouth and nose
    4. Vomiting
    5. Urine
    6. Feces
  C. Investigation
    1. More prevalent in murdering of infants than adults
    2. In killing of young infants merely hand may be used
    3. In the killing of adults
        a. Search for signs of struggle
        b. Implements used, such as pillow, etc.

V. Gagging and choking
    A. When nose and mouth obstructed by cloth or the like tied around head
        OR
    B. Placed in mouth
        1. Obstructing pharynx
          or
        2. Forcing tongue against fauces, causing complete obstruction to respiration
    C. Choking
        1. Solid objects or materials enter and obstruct air passages
          (Usually accidental)
        2. Sometimes death may not result immediately (obstruction not complete)
          Sometimes vagal shock
        3. Also may be caused by regurgitation of food
          a. Drunks
          b. Infants
          c. Elderly persons
        4. Features
          a. Face cyanosed, and
          b. Sometimes swollen
          c. Face and eyes—petechial hemorrhages
          d. Tongue swollen
          e. Foreign body may be observed in mouth and throat

VI. Traumatic
    A. External pressure to chest and abdomen, arresting respiratory movements
    B. Appearances
        1. Purplish, black cyanosis of face and neck

    2. Petechial hemorrhage of face, chest, shoulders and neck

VII. Chemicals

    A. Household ammonia, ether, chloroform, sulpha dioxide, etcetera

    B. Breathing of these fumes in high concentration may become so irritating that paralysis of respiration occurs

VIII. Drowning

    See Chapter on Drowning

—24—

ARSON AND OTHER FIRES
SYNOPSIS

Fires of incendiary origin may be started: (1) accidentally; (2) by persons seeking to defraud insurance companies; (3) by persons seeking to conceal a suicidal or homicidal death; (4) as a result of a prank; (5) from persons who are of a psychotic nature; or (6) as a means of homicide itself.

Careful investigation is necessary to reveal and to determine: (1) the cause of death; (2) possible cover-up of a crime; (3) type of inflammable material used; (4) identification of dead bodies; (5) cause and manner of all deaths; (6) if more than one person, sequence of death; and (7) exact role of fire and cause of death.

Most conflagration deaths are caused through accidental means and are frequently caused from invalidity and semi-consciousness caused through the use of drugs and alcohol. Careful examination of the bodies and of the scene is very important in discovering significant clues. Identification of dead persons is extremely difficult, and evidence used in this identification is often fragmentary. Extreme care should be exercised in the determination of the identification of particular bones or parts of bodies as to: (1) whether they are human or animal, and (2) as to the exact individual to whom they belonged.

Releases on possible identification, sex, age, etc., should await examination by anthropologist, orthopedist and autopsy by pathologist.

Even if the subject is buried in lye or other caustic agents, or burned in the extreme heat of a furnace, the saving of all the debris, and the sifting and saving of all the ashes, might well give the expert the important clue that the investigator can then use to answer his questions and solve his case.

The investigator should remember that, although most conflagrations are accidental in nature, they may also be used either to commit or to conceal a crime; however, he should also remember that very seldom, if ever, does a fire destroy all clues.

(Form 17—Body Burn Percentage Chart)

ARSON AND OTHER FIRES

I. General—types of fires most frequently occurring
   A. Arson
      1. The intentional and illegal burning of a dwelling or out-house, or other type building, as defined by Statutes of respective states
      2. Usually a felony, with different degrees of arson, depending on type of building burned and under what circumstances
      3. At Common Law punishable by death
      4. Under Statutory Law may be murder, if death results therefrom
   B. Careless smoking or careless use of matches
   C. Defective overheated heating or cooking equipment
   D. Defective electrical equipment
   E. Careless use of inflammable liquids
   F. Defective chimneys or flues
II. Injury to subject
   A. Categories of burning
      1. Causative agent (heat, electricity, chemicals, radiation, etc.)
      2. Severity (1st, 2nd, 3rd and 4th degrees)
      3. Extent (portion of body affected)
   B. Severity
      1. 1st degree—redness
      2. 2nd degree—vesication (blistering)

      3. 3rd degree—damage to fat, muscle, tis-
         sues and even bare bone

      4. 4th degree—charring

  C. Extent (method of approximate estimation)
      1. Head 6%
      2. Upper extremities 18%
      3. Trunk 38%
      4. Lower extremities 38%

Note: Where 50% or more of the body is burned,
the result is usually fatal, regardless of which
parts are affected

  D. Burning may cause
      1. Bleeding
      2. Fractures

Note: Fractures may occur by contraction and by
fire itself

  E. Injuries
      1. Blistering
      2. Acute pain
      3. Shock
      4. Toxemia
      5. Infections
      6. Carbon monoxide poisoning
         a. One may have some carbon monoxide
           by taking only one breath
         b. Carbon monoxide content must be de-
           termined by blood test
         c. Where subject has a large amount of
           carbon monoxide, may be seen by
           "cherry red" lividity and also by "cher-
           ry red" color of blood
      7. Nerve reflex

III. Questions to be answered
  A. Did death occur before, after or during fire?

      B.   Cause of death

      C.   Identification of body

      D.   Contributing factors

          1. Alcohol

          2. Drugs

          3. Injuries

          4. Natural diseases

      E.   Manner of death

          1. Accident

          2. Suicide

          3. Homicide

          4. Natural

IV.   Proof that subject was alive during fire

      A.   Smoke and soot in air passages

      B.   Carbon monoxide in blood

      C.   Reddening at the edge of the burns, indicating active circulation of the blood

      D.   Tissue fluids present in the blisters

      E.   Skull fracture (?)

          1. Skull fracture from heat usually creates a straight fracture line with expansion from within causing bursting to the outside

          2. Skull fracture from a blow usually creates a radiating line with hemorrhage damage to the brain underneath

      F.   Splits in skin will not bleed if the subject is dead at the time of being exposed to the heat

V.   Causes of death

      A.   Falling objects

      B.   Excessive heat

      C.   Anoxia (lack of oxygen)

D. Noxious gases (Carbon Monoxide, Carbon Dioxide, etc.)
E. Delayed deaths
   1. Edema
   2. Shock
   3. Pneumonia
   4. Infection
VI. Investigation (Fig. 43 and Fig. 44)
   A. Determining point of origin of fire
      1. Ceiling
         Heat rises, and may therefore locate start of fire by concentration of greatest burning point at ceiling
      2. Metal
         Will become twisted and distorted by longest application of heat

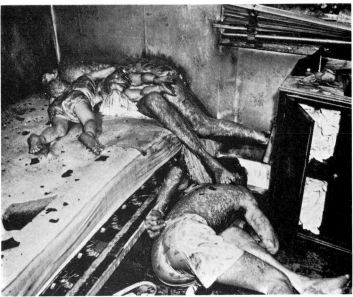

FIG. 43. Fire. Death by carbon monoxide poisoning.

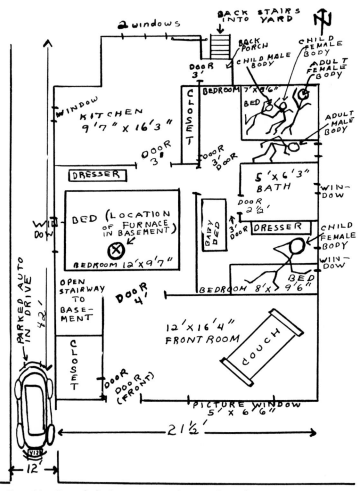

Fɪɢ. 44. Detailed diagraming of preceding figure.

3. Wood
    Point of deepest charring of wood
4. Walls
    Point of heaviest concentration of smoke
    or greatest burning

    5. Insulation on electric wires destroyed
    6. Floors
     Charring or burning
VII. Evidence
  A. Mechanical and electrical devices
    1. Retain all devices
    2. Deliver to laboratory intact
    3. When connected to explosives, protect and leave undisturbed for dismantling by experts
  B. Paper (streamers, wastepaper, etc.)
    1. Retain all
    2. If saturated with gasoline or other flammable materials, pack in clean glass container with tight cover
    3. If dry, pack in box
  C. Wood
    1. Retain all
    2. Pack in clean, individual wrappers or dry glass containers
  D. Chemicals and liquids
    1. Retain all to maximum of one quart
    2. Store in dry, sterile glass containers with tight covers
  E. Kerosene and gasoline
    1. Retain all
    2. Store in dry, sterile glass containers with tight covers
  F. Solids
    1. Retain all to maximum of one pound
    2. Store in clean, individual wrappers, or dry glass containers
  G. Ashes (Fig. 45)

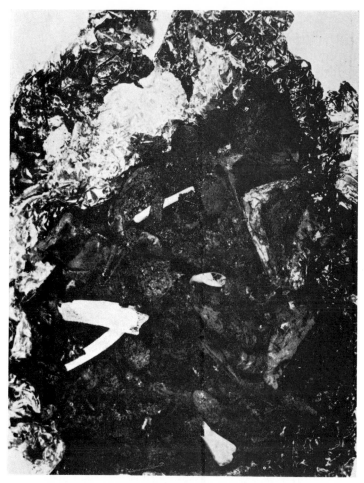

Fɪɢ. 45.   Bones recovered in arson preserved by aluminum foil.

1. Retain samples from different portions of premises and all different types of items within premises
2. Store in clean glass containers with tight lids

H. Explosives or bombs
    Consult expert for recommendations and
    manner of removal
I. Lye and other strong basis
    Store in glass container with glass stoppers
J. Bones or skeleton material (Fig. 46)
    1. Wrap separately in paper, soft cotton
        cloth or cotton padding
    2. Store in carton filled with cotton waste
        or rags

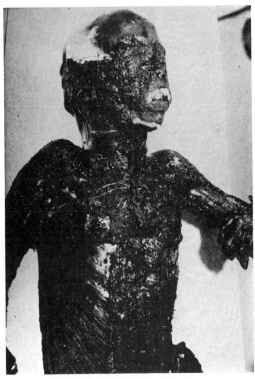

Fig. 46. Entire destruction of features by burning.

  K.   Glass fragments
       1. Collect all particles and fragments
       2. Wrap each piece individually in cotton
           or soft paper
       3. Store rigidly in a box
       4. Protect all stains
       5. Submit for comparison with any glass
           suspected of being identical
VIII. Cause of fire
  A.   Consult experts
       1. Fire Department
       2. Electrical experts
       3. Gas experts
       4. Chemical experts

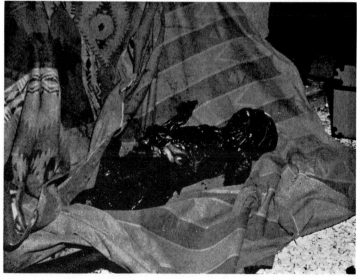

Fig. 47. Death by burning, showing bursting of skin due to heat.

B. Witnesses
1. As to approximate time flame or smoke first seen
2. As to location of possible point of origin
3. As to possible suspects or persons seen in or about the premises
4. As to possible deficiencies in electrical or other appliances and connections

(Fig. 47)

—25—

AUTOMOBILE FATALITIES
SYNOPSIS

When a crime is committed with a lethal weapon such as a gun or knife, a great deal of time and care is taken by the investigators to secure every bit of information necessary to determine the identity of and to convict the wrongdoer; however, when the weapon used is an automobile, the investigation seems to take on a less important atmosphere, thereby becoming more lax and incomplete. Because of the investigator's attitude, coupled with the fact that he usually lacks proper equipment, the relevant laws are insufficient to properly deal with the violations and that the average citizen fails to cooperate, the obviously guilty life taker is allowed to go free with little or no punishment although he has committed one of the greatest sins against nature and against the law—that of wrongly depriving somebody else of his life.

It is extremely unfortunate that killing by an automobile is one of the very few ways that one can literally commit murder and avoid the law, and it is unfortunate that those people who have committed that serious crime of taking another human's life and are responsible both criminally and morally for that fatality can, firstly, go free, and secondly, are not even deprived of the use of that instrument with which that crime was committed.

It is estimated that less than ten percent of those drivers who have taken a life as a result of or during a violation of the law either go free entirely or receive punishment that is not in the least in proportion to the severity of the crime committed.

Death as the result of a motor vehicle collision can be classified in the following categories: accident, negligent, careless and reckless, manslaughter, justifiable homicide, murder in the second degree, or murder in the first degree; for criminal investigation the coroner and law enforcement officers are principally interested in three of these categories, to-wit: accident, careless and reckless, or manslaughter.

Preliminary detailed and accurate investigating of an automobile fatality and correctly and completely reporting of same are indispensable in bringing about prosecution and eventual conviction.

It is often stated that a picture is worth a thousand words and this is especially true in the matter of automobile fatalities. It is recommended that all policemen and law enforcement officials carry simple type cameras in their automobiles, which cameras will allow them to photograph the scene of automobile collisions so that the same will be clear to them as well as to those to whom they later describe what was seen and occurred. Also, it is often true in the study of a picture that it may reveal something that the eye or the eye witnesses overlooked. Close-ups are not necessary because of the difficulty in taking same clearly and because the developer can "blow up" a scene to bring out details. Colored photographs, although not always admissible in a court trial, are advisable for more careful observation and study of details.

Whether or not a camera is used, a complete diagram of the road, intersections, automobiles, bodies and other evidence should be made, measuring distance either by tape measure or paces, and locating the exact scene of the impact by direction and distance from an identifiable point.

(This preliminary diagram should be preserved, and a more complete and detailed one prepared at the office.) (Fig. 48)

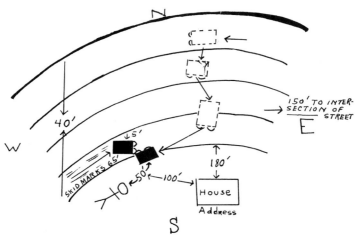

FIG. 48. Sketching of scene.

Skid marks and debris on the highway should be collected before persons or vehicles can contaminate, destroy or move same.

At that point the automobiles may be moved to the side of the road and traffic allowed to pass.

Although the automobiles have then been moved to the side of the road they should not be removed from the scene itself until a check is made and samples taken of: (1) contents in the car, (2) blood stains in and about the car, (3) worn paint, (4) broken doors or glass (in order to perhaps trace the sources of injuries), (5) operating condition of the car, especially the brakes and the lights, (6) engine and serial number and license number, (7) pictures wherever possible, and until (8) the coroner's office is informed. Any evidence found during the search should be identified by the officer, initialed and placed in a bag or box, or wrapped up and kept in the officer's possession. Where evidence may be pieces of metal or wood or glass, the officer should attempt to scratch his initial or some identifying mark on that piece of evidence; this can be done with a knife, key or any sharp instrument.

While one officer is accomplishing or attempting to accomplish all the above, another officer should determine the exact location of the wounded and dead and should obtain the names and addresses of all witnesses. He should determine from these witnesses certain basic points regarding the time and place of the accident, the direction of the vehicles, their approximate speed, and all other information that the witnesses can give him.

The officer at that time should attempt to establish the identity of the drivers of the vehicles and their passengers, and should attempt to obtain at least a limited statement from them embracing certain important elements, for example: the time of the accident, liquor consumption (including liquor tests if possible), ownership of the vehicles, operating conditions of the vehicles, where they were coming from, where they were going, approximate time of the accident, any driving restrictions that the operators may have had, previous violations, driving experience, familiarity with road and driving conditions on that road, and a short description as to what happened. Statements, however short, should be written by the officer in the exact words of the witnesses, dated and signed by the witnesses.

A written record should be made at the time regarding the condition of the weather, the visibility at the time, blind spots on the road, hills and curves in the vicinity, speed limit, stop signs and other signs, condition of the road, material of which road is made, lighting, width of the highway, number of lanes in the highway, closest intersection, and how many previous collisions occurred at that particular locale. This history is not only helpful in determining what happened in this collision, but in the making of any recommendation to avoid such future collisions.

The above type of investigation is also recommended in the case of leaving the scene, or a hit and run type of collision, with particular emphasis being placed upon the investigation, examination and interrogation of the witnesses, and determining the exact description of the automobile involved. Any type of debris or other physical evidence, no matter how seemingly small, may make or break the case.

Where there is a fatality involved, the operators of each of the vehicles involved in that fatality should be apprehended and placed under arrest on suspicion of committing the felony of manslaughter, and should not be re-released without some kind of bond. An investigating officer should not himself attempt to determine whether criminal prosecution should be had.

It is also recommended that the investigating officer then recommend to the drivers of the various vehicles that they submit to an alcoholic test.

(Form 18—Vehicle Stopping Distance Chart)
(Form 26—Auto Accident Report)

AUTOMOBILE FATALITIES

I. General
  A. Injuries inflicted to pedestrian victim (Fig. 49)
    1. Vehicle striking victim
    2. Victim striking ground or other object
    3. Vehicle running over part of victim
    4. Complications resulting from injuries
  B. Usual injuries
    1. Bumper injuries
    2. Contact of subject with ground
      a. Usually head
      b. Abrasions, bruises and lacerations to other parts
    3. Injuries from car running over subject, which depends on
      a. The part of body run over
      b. Weight of vehicle
      c. Speed of vehicle
      d. Nature of ground underneath (whether hard or soft, etc.)

II. Investigation
  A. Scene
    1. If accident appears of a serious nature, officers should radio for help, in that no one officer is capable of completely handling and reporting a serious automobile accident

161

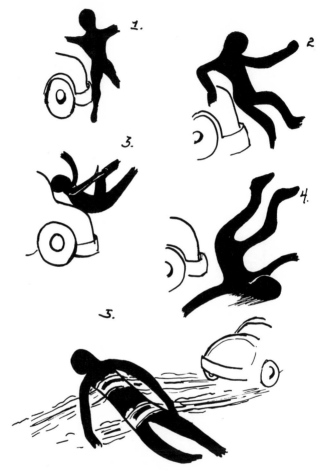

FIG. 49. Illustration indicating injuries to pedestrian
(a) Vehicle striking victim.
(b) and (c) Victim striking vehicle after initial impact.
(d) Victim striking ground.
(e) Victim being run over by vehicle.

2. Traffic should be stopped or detoured momentarily, so that road scene is not destroyed
3. Witnesses should be detained for later identification and questioning
4. Measurements and rough drawings should be made
5. Pictures taken
6. Tire marks and angles thereof noted
7. Skid marks
   a. Location
   b. Length
   c. Direction
   d. Particular beginning and ending points
8. Debris on highway
   a. To establish exact point of impact
   b. To establish identity of vehicles
   c. To establish directions of car, where traveling
   d. To establish directions and angle cars traveled after collision
9. Pictures taken (Fig. 50)
   a. In a clockwise direction
   b. Of the road and parts of road involved
   c. Of the place of impact
   d. Of the distances and place of skids
   e. Of direction of the automobiles after impact
   f. Of the place where the automobiles came to rest
   g. Of the automobiles themselves

B. Of the automobile
   1. Contents in the automobile

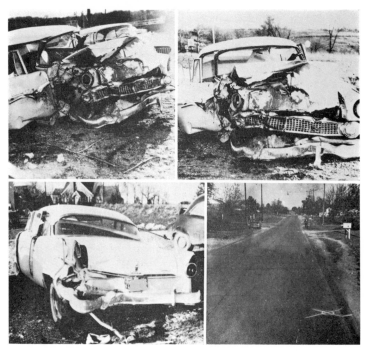

Fig. 50. Correct way to photograph automobile to show damage and identification of automobile; photographing of scene after automobile is removed.

2. Blood stains in and about the car
   a. May be flaked off and placed in pill boxes
   b. Use different blades of knife to remove separate samples (single edge razor blade suggested)
   c. Wet paint should be placed in glass bottles
   Note: Blood samples very important in hit and run cases

3. Worn paint
4. Foreign paint
   Samples taken in same manner as blood
5. Broken doors and glass (in order to trace the sources of injury)
6. Operating condition of the car, especially
   a. Brakes
   b. Lights
7. Engine, serial and license numbers
8. Dirt from underneath fenders
9. Oil
10. Tire marks (Fig. 51)
11. Material obviously coming from automobile
12. Marks of victim on car
    a. Glass
    b. Blood
    c. Clothing
    d. Fibers
    e. Particles of skin

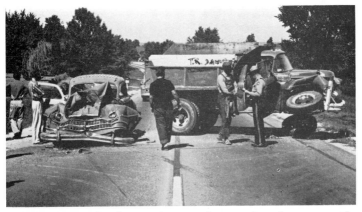

Fig. 51 Tire marks showing how truck crossed to the wrong side of the road before striking vehicle head-on.

13. Pictures
    a. Front view
    b. Left side
    c. Right side
    d. Rear
    e. Pictures should identify automobile and where possible show license plate
    f. Bottom of automobile, especially where pedestrian run over
14. Other evidence to be taken by officer
    a. Entire automobile
       OR
    b. Part of automobile showing collision
    Note: Officer should not hesitate to take an entire fender or bumper where necessary to prove hit and run case
C. Of victim (Fig. 52)
    1. Marks on victim
       a. Glass
       b. Paint
       c. Radiator or other vehicle pattern
       d. Metal
       e. Tire
       f. Measure imprint or wound on victim from the sole up, so as to identify same as being from a particular part of the automobile of the same height above the ground (Fig. 53).
    2. Clothing of victim should be carefully preserved to transmit to laboratory for tests for
       a. Paint
       b. Pieces of metal
       c. Possible tears

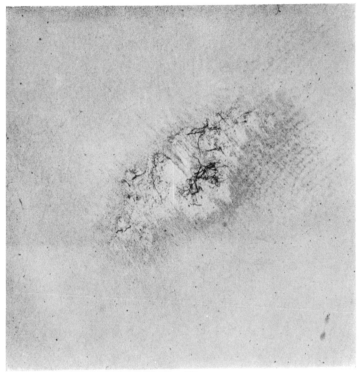

Fig. 52a

FIG. 52. (a) Fabric of clothing with fibers; (b) Position of initial impact; (c) Type of wound; and (d) Comparing with damage to hit and run vehicle—all of which established identity of vehicle and guilt of hit and run driver.

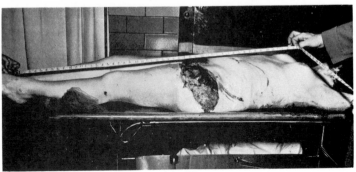

Fig. 52b

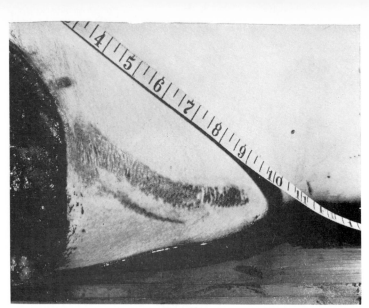

Fig. 52c

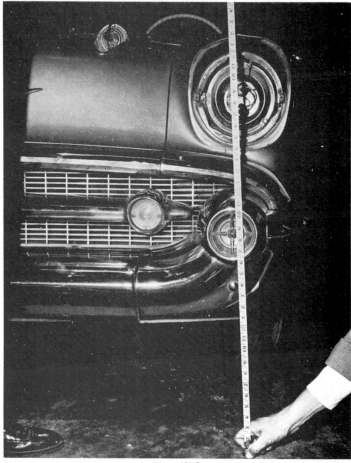

Fig. 52d

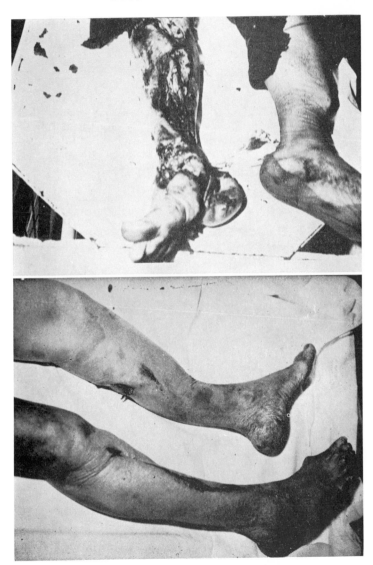

FIG. 53. Pedestrians struck by auto—bumper fractures.

        d. Dirt from highway or automobile

        e. Oil or grease from highway or auto-mobile

        f. Alcoholic content

D.   Of driver or drivers

      1. Sobriety (alcohol test)

      2. Should be questioned on the scene of facts surrounding the accident
         AND

      3. Movements immediately preceding the accident

  Note: Questioning at the scene necessary for "res gestae"

E.   Other facts to be noted

      1. Condition of weather

      2. Visibility at time

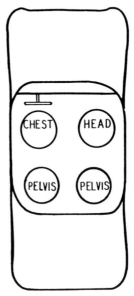

Fig. 54. Usual injury to occupants of automobile collision

3. Blind spots on roads
4. Hills and curves in vicinity
5. Speed limit
6. Stop signs and other signs
7. Material of which road is made
8. Lighting conditions
9. Width of highway
10. Number of lanes
11. Nearest intersection
12. Names and addresses of all witnesses
    a. Witnesses to the collision
    b. Witnesses to the manner in which the vehicle was operating immediately prior to the collision

(Fig. 54)

-26-

BLUNT IMPACT
SYNOPSIS

Blunt impact, or crushing blow to the head, is a method sometimes used to conceal a homicide. The manner of so concealing this homicide can usually be accomplished by throwing the subject down a long flight of steps or dropping a heavy weight on him, after he has been struck, thereby creating an appearance of an accident. Thusly, the investigation of anyone who has died of head injuries by allegedly falling down the steps or having a heavy object fall on him, should be conducted with the thought of determining whether the fatal blow was from the fall or from an object at the hands of a person delivered prior to that fall.

A careful search should be made throughout the entire house and adjacent grounds for weapons, stones, bricks or heavy pieces of wood (usually 2" x 4") that could have been used, at the same time looking for blood and other stains and any signs of a struggle. In searching for the weapon or means of crushing, it should be noted that the wound is not usually the same size or shape as the murder instrument. However, the instrument used may show something, e.g., stains, a strand of hair, a dent, and, therefore, should be handled carefully so as not to destroy the evidence or smudge the palm prints or fingerprints that may be on it.

In such cases, the investigator should take complete pictures, indicating the position of the body in relation to the steps, to the walls and to any object that could have accounted for the wounds. Pictures should also show the number and type of steps and should be taken looking up and looking down the steps.

The type of doors at the top of the steps, the manner (in or out) in which they open, the lighting, the hallway or room leading to the steps, the possibility of mistaking the entrance to the steps with another entrance, where the subject was apparently going or from where he was coming—all facts should be investigated to determine if the alleged fall at that particular time could have been accidental.

The condition of the clothing, blood stains on the steps or floor, angle of the body, position of the head (in placing the subject on the floor to "show accident" the murderer might not realize that oftentimes when one is struck on one side of the head, the other side is damaged and hemorrhages; this is called "contrecoup"); also, the number of fractures or external wounds might indicate that the subject was struck before he was thrown down the steps. Particles of hairs on wood steps, splinters from wooden steps—all these are important in distinguishing between accident and murder.

Alcohol tests later prove important to determine the subject's condition and reflexes at the time, in that the majority of accidental falls are suffered by "drunks"; a large number are caused by dark hallways late at night with the doors leading to the basement and to the bathroom being close together.

Suspicion in these cases is the keynote to a thorough and complete investigation. It should be remembered in the investigation, and in the later questioning of the relatives and friends who were on the premises, that the closer the relationship the easier to commit the homicide and hide the deed.

BLUNT IMPACT

Definition: Injury by agent which is neither of a penetrating nor cutting nature

I. Wounds—General
   A. Depends on
      1. Nature of agent responsible
      2. Force and angle
      3. Mobility of part of body struck
      4. Area of body struck
      5. Physique of victim
   B. Falls—Injury depends on
      1. Force of fall
      2. Surface on which body falls
      3. Parts of body which strike surface
      4. Whether that part of the body is clothed
      Note: Usually accidental or following attack due to natural causes
   C. Types
      1. Abrasions (Fig. 55 and Fig. 56)
      2. Contusions
      3. Lacerations
      Note: All three types may be on the same wound
   D. Injuries to head
      1. Contrecoup (Fig. 57)
         Damage on side opposite to that struck by blow
      2. Direct impact
      3. Delayed death—rupture of arteries supplying membranes that cover the brain—

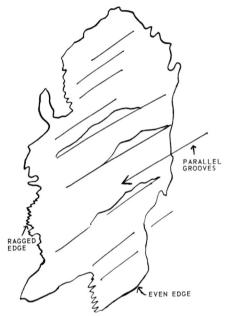

FIG. 55. Abrasion showing direction of force.

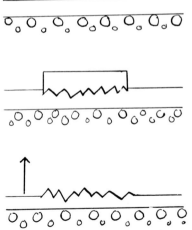

FIG. 56. Illustration showing abrasion wound caused by rubbing
surface of skin with a rough object.

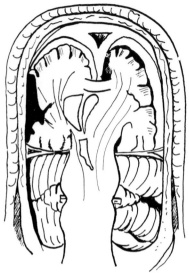

FIG. 57. Contrecoup. Note brain actually striking skull on the left side of the head; original blow was to the right side of the head; damage created by pressure.

   meninges (slow oozing—until large clot is formed)
  4. Subdural hematoma (Fig. 58)
 II. Abrasions
  A. Generally
   1. Mostly superficial
   2. Damage to outer layer of skin only
   3. Not dangerous to life itself
   4. Important for evidence
    a. Movement and pressure by agent on surface of skin are necessary for abrasions
    b. Pressure depends on
     (1) Roughness of agent in contact with skin

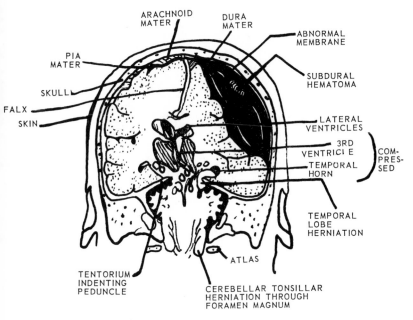

Fig. 58. Subdural hematoma.

        (2) Velocity
        (3) Pressure
            (Example: ligature around neck)
   B.   Important in investigation to show
      1. Only external sign of injury
      2. Site of external impact
      3. Impression of instrument
         (pressure abrasion)
   C.   When (subject alive or dead)
      1. Life—dries up and becomes a scab
      2. After death
        a. Shortly after—yellow parchment
        b. Sometime after — post-mortem discoloration

Difference must be determined by microscopic examination

D. Kinds
1. Sliding or scraping abrasions (scratch)
   a. Occurs—movement between skin and rough object
   b. Can tell direction and responsible agent
   c. Falls—conscious person will use hands —abrasions on hands or fingers
2. Pressure or crushing abrasions
   a. Movement necessary
   b. Movement slight and directed inwards —crushing superficial layer of the cuticle

Note: Fingernail abrasions may be usually seen in sexual assaults

3. Contusions or bruises
   a. Rupture of blood vessels (usually capillaries)
      Occurs more readily in young persons
   b. Color
      (1) Fresh bruise
          Dark red or purple — uniform in color
      (2) After 24 hours
          Lighter margin
      (3) After few days
          Changes to green and yellow
   c. May last weeks or months
   d. Evidence
      (1) Size — does not usually indicate size of instrument causing it

       (2) May become visible days after injury

       (3) May appear away from actual site of blow

       (4) May be inflicted a short period after death

III. Lacerations

    A. Definition: Split or tear of the skin

       1. Caused
          By a crushing or shearing force
          Usually over bony prominences

       2. Bruising
          a. Extent depends on force of blow
            AND
          b. What area of skin actually touched

    B. Must be distinguished from incised wounds

       1. Lacerations usually occur over bony prominences
          whereas
          Incised wounds occur any place on body

       2. Lacerations create wounds which are irregular, with bruising on edge of wounds
          whereas
          Incised wounds are straight and clean-cut, with no bruising

       3. Laceration usually creates minimal bleeding
          whereas
          Incised wounds cause great bleeding

       4. Lacerations affect usually soft structures which become torn
          whereas
          Incised wounds will neatly divide to extreme depth of wound

5. Lacerations usually contain foreign bodies, such as fibers of clothing
whereas
Incised wounds are free from foreign body

6. Lacerations are usually accidental (example: falls),
whereas
Incised wounds are usually caused intentionally

7. BOTH lacerations and incised wounds of the scalp or head usually bleed profusely, even when inflicted after death

IV. Notes
    A.   One blow
       Although big laceration is caused, there may be no blood on instrument or coming from the wound.
    Note: Blood expelled from tissues beneath the site of the blow
    B.   More than one blow (Fig. 59)
       1. Will force blood through torn vessels under pressure
         AND
       2. Project it in all directions and for a distance
    C.   Appearance of spurted blood
       Exclamation mark — pointed away from bleeding
       1. Arterial spurting—one direction and regular
       2. Lacerated spurting — all directions
    D.   Examination of blood
       1. Pools — where lying

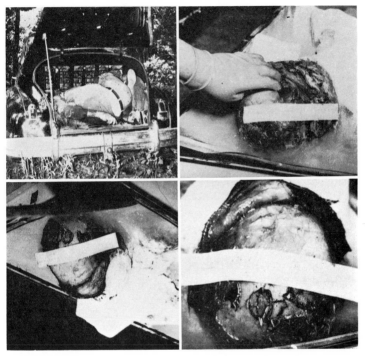

Fig. 59. Death by crushing; subject struck on head by blunt object and then stuffed in trunk of automobile.

2. Stains on clothing to indicate the position of the body at and after the blow
3. Instruments
    a. May have blood, hair, fibers or prints
    b. When a sharp metal instrument is used, creating incised wound, little or no blood will adhere to the metal blade

—27—

CARBON MONOXIDE
SYNOPSIS

Death from carbon monoxide usually results from an accident or from a desire of suicide. Only careful investigation of the scene will determine whether it is either of these or whether the death was caused by homicide.

In addition to determining what agents were responsible for causing the death, it is often necessary to decide exactly when and how the subject died. This is particularly true in cases of fire to discover whether the deceased expired as the result of burning or as a result of the smoke created by the fire. Another possibility is that the subject was murdered prior to the fire itself, which was set to conceal the homicide.

Snap decisions at the scene can easily lead to a relaxing of the investigation, and a premature news release, which might be wrong, could easily cause the investigator a great deal of embarrassment and chagrin.

It is of utmost importance, therefore, to preserve the scene and the evidence therein until such time that an autopsy is performed and blood tests taken and analyzed.

Sometimes lividity resembling the color caused by carbon monoxide may be seen on the subject, but here again careful investigation of the scene and autopsy are very important. This misleading lividity can be caused through a heart attack, consumption of some types of poisons, and asphyxia by certain chemicals commonly used around the house or shop, such as ammonia, ether, chloroform and sulphur dioxide.

(Form 23—Carbon Monoxide Report)

CARBON MONOXIDE

I. General characteristics
   A. Colorless
   B. May be odorless
   C. Lighter than air
II. Sources
   A. Coal gas
   B. Natural gases
   C. Heat
   D. Car exhaust
      1. Approximately 50% of carbon monoxide in exhaust after car runs for a few minutes
      2. Unconsciousness will result in approximately five minutes
   E. Fires
   F. Smoke
III. Effect on body
   A. Not poisonous per se, but may be when
      1. Anemic anoxia is caused by reduction of oxy-hemoglobin available for respiration AND/OR
      2. The excretion of carbon dioxide is interfered with
   B. Concentration of over 40% in blood stream is almost always fatal, this amount depending on
      1. Amount in atmosphere
      2. Respiratory rate

        3. Area temperature and humidity

        4. Oxygen content

        5. Amount of other gases in atmosphere

        6. Rate of oxygen disassociation

        7. Presence or absence of pre-existing causes of anoxia

    C. Carbon monoxide affects

        1. Cardiovascular system

        AND

        2. Central nervous system

    D. Symptoms

        1. Dizziness

        2. Drowsiness

        3. Headache

        4. Nausea

        5. Confusion

        6. Impaired judgment

        7. Reflexes

        8. Vomiting

        9. Coma

IV. Investigation of body (Fig. 60)

    A. Body is usually cherry red in color

        BUT

    B. Cherry red patches may appear on skin when the death is delayed

    Note: Death is not always instantaneous

    C. No redness where subject has been bleeding profusely

    D. No redness where bodies are extensively burned

    Note: Chemical analysis of the blood is necessary to determine presence and extent of carbon monoxide poisoning (Fig. 61)

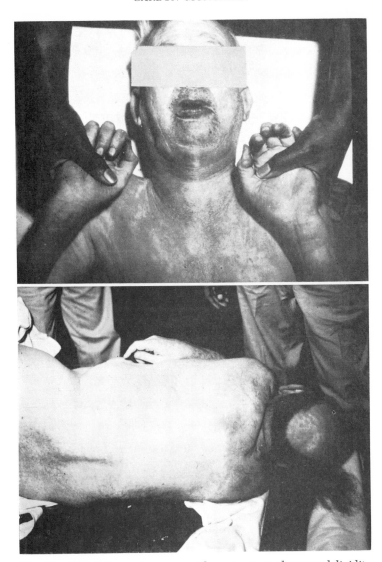

Fig. 60. Death by carbon monoxide poisoning; cherry red lividity in shoulders and face. Note previous suicide attempts—semi-healed slashes on wrist.

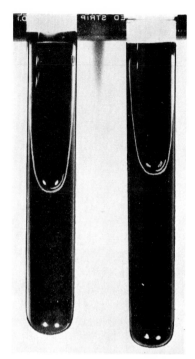

Fig. 61 Death by carbon monoxide poisoning. Note lighter shade of blood on the left (carbon monoxide), which is actually cherry red, as compared to darker blood on the right (natural death).

V. Investigation of scene
  A. Building or garage
    1. Entire dimensions (cubic area)
    2. Open or closed condition of doors, windows and other apertures
    3. Open gas outlets
    4. Faulty heating and cooking equipment
    5. Position of body
    6. Notes
    7. Indication of foul play

    8. Odor of gas
    9. Apertures sealed, and how
  10. Ventilators and flues
  11. Meters

B.   Automobile
    1. If in a garage whether door and windows are closed
    2. Whether windows and doors of automobile are closed
    3. Hose or other equipment attached to exhaust
      a. How attached
      b. Where obtained
      c. How exhaust fed into automobile
    4. Whether ignition of automobile on or off
    5. Whether motor is running
      a. How gas pedal is held down
      b. How much gasoline in car
      c. If motor not running
        (1) Whether motor warm or cold
        Note: Comparative warmth of motor may help determine time of death
        (2) Whether motor could have died by itself
    6. Whether subject sitting or lying on the seat until death resulted

—28—

DROWNING

SYNOPSIS

Death by drowning is usually accidental, except in the case of infants who are killed by drowning much more numerously than are adults. Contrary to some belief, it is possible to commit suicide by drowning.

Also contrary to some belief, many "drownings" are not in reality death caused by drowning, but the result of a swimmer having succumbed to a natural cause while in the process of swimming, the most common of these being a coronary or heart condition.

Usually when a person dies by drowning, there is evidence of foam coming out of the nose and the mouth (which is usually open), bluish appearance of the body (especially in cold water) and lividity in the face and neck. Final conclusion must be left to the pathologist after autopsy.

When a body has sunk to the bottom of the water it will rise after a period of time (not 3 times as is commonly believed), unless it is restricted to the bottom because of being stuck to foreign objects or as the result of having been weighted down by foreign objects or because of the condition of the water itself. The body is able to rise to the top because of the formation of gases in the body tissue and putrefaction.

The amount of putrefaction, destruction of tissues and skin, stenches, lack of clothing and hair (lost in water or eaten by fish), etcetera, are clues as to approximate time of death. Bruises could indicate if the subject struck an object, then lost consciousness and died as a result of striking that object, or as result of drowning.

Identification is very difficult in these cases. The body should be left undisturbed until examination by the expert in order to eliminate the risk of destroying important marks on the body or of tearing any loosened skin or tissue from the body.

Search for a drowned body is very difficult and should be undertaken only after consultation with expert on river to determine current, depth and the like, so as not to waste time needlessly or to risk lives unnecessarily.

DROWNING

I. General
   A. Death resulting from drowning is usually due to asphyxia
   B. "Dry" drowning
      1. Subject swallows quantity of water
      2. Water found in stomach
   C. "Wet" drowning
      1. Water found in trachea
   D. Quantity of water very seldom found in lungs even though death may be due to drowning

II. Time of rising of body
   A. Human body will sink in fresh water (body heavier than air)
   B. Body will usually rise to surface
      1. Due to gas formation because of decay and putrefaction
      2. Time of rising depends on
         a. Depth of water
         b. Temperature of water
         c. Whether body entangled in rocks or weeds
         d. Currents

III. Signs on body (Fig. 62 and Fig 63)
   A. White foam from nose and mouth
   B. Objects in hand—grass, mud, etcetera
   C. Cadaveric spasm of both hands
      (caused by subject frantically clutching for something at time of drowning)

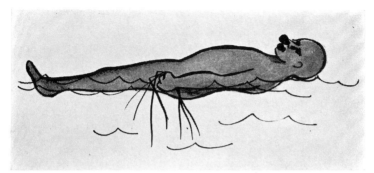

Fig. 62. Death by drowning; bubbles from nostrils and mouth, and weeds in clenched hand.

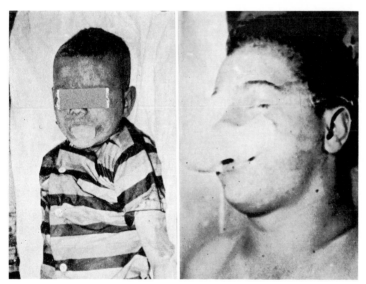

Fig. 63. Death by drowning; bubbles from nostrils and mouth.

D. Fingernail marks on palm of hand
E. Post-mortem lividity in head and neck
F. Mouth usually open
G. Petechial spots in eyes

IV. Identification of body
   A. After period of time in water skin becomes very loose and extreme care in handling of body must be exercised so as not to destroy evidence
   B. Skin may be destroyed by
      1. Being eaten by fish
      2. Putrefaction (Fig. 64)
      3. Decay

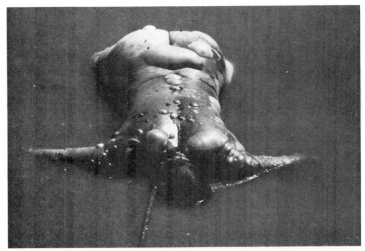

FIG. 64. Death by drowning. Note putrefaction blisters forming after being in water forty-eight hours in summertime.

   C. Modes of identification
      1. Teeth
      2. Clothing on body
      3. Fingerprints
         a. First attempt to take fingerprints in normal manner
         b. Sometimes hands may be clean and fingerprints taken by photographer

    c. Skin may be built up by saline and other solutions

    d. Skin may be stripped and sent to laboratories

        (1) Stripping should be done by pathologist

        (2) Extreme care must be exercised to remove skin on entire distal joint

        (3) Prepare 10 bottles with preservative solution

        (4) Mark each bottle, designating finger and hand (e.g., thumb, right hand, etc.)

        (5) As skin is removed, place in appropriate bottle and seal

  4. Hair

  5. Operative scars

  Note: Because of condition of body may oftentimes have to be determined by x-ray or autopsy

V. Autopsy to determine

  A. Whether death actually due from drowning

  B. Possible wounds inflicted before drowning

  C. Probable time of death

  Note: Drownings are usually accidental

  Note: After subject has been in water a period of time decay and putrefaction of body tissues make determination of cause of death very difficult even on autopsy—collateral investigation of physical circumstances very important

  Note: Body does NOT go down three times before death finally occurs

—29—

ELECTROCUTION

SYNOPSIS

Most deaths caused by electrocution are accidental in nature.

In order for a person to be electrocuted, one part of him must touch the conductor and another must be grounded. Thusly, in examining a person for electrocution one must necessarily search for a point of entry and a point of exit. It is possible for a person to have been electrocuted even though there are no visible burn signs on the outer skin, and evidence of the electrocution must be determined by autopsy.

Contrariwise, the body may be almost totally consumed by the flame and heat.

The investigator should also remember that when a person is apparently electrocuted there may be indications of lack of breathing, eye changes and other signs of death when, in effect, he is actually in a state of shock or coma. When the investigator is confronted with such a situation, artificial respiration and/or an inhalator should be applied until such time that he is actually pronounced dead by a physician or until rigor mortis has definitely set in.

Death from lightning is a type of electrocution, and will oftentimes also indicate points of entrance and exit.

ELECTROCUTION

I. General
   A. Effect on body
      1. Central nervous system
      2. Cardiovascular (pertaining to the heart and blood vessels)
      3. Burning
      4. Asphyxia due to spasm of respiratory muscles
   B. Important elements
      1. Voltage (tension of charge)
      2. Amperage (intensity)
      3. Ground
   Note: In order for subject to be electrocuted he must have contact with live wire and must be grounded
   C. Conductor and resistance
      1. Dry skin—bad conductor
      2. Thickened area (hands, fingers, soles of feet)—bad conductor
      3. Moisture—lowers resistance
II. External signs
   A. Electrical burns at entrance and exit (Fig. 65)
   B. Entrance
      1. Disruption of tissues
      2. Steam liberated from dampness and water in system
      3. Pattern of electrical object usually reproduced on skin—sometimes zigzag
   C. Flash in sparkle—widespread burning

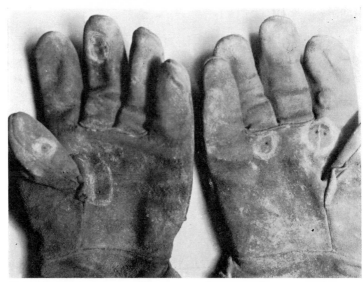

Fɪɢ. 65. Electrocution. Entrance and exit marks.

    D.   Metal on skin acts as conductor, creating burn underneath

    E.   Possible rigor mortis appearing immediately

III.   Investigation—scene

    A.   Contact and ground

    B.   Live wire

    C.   Proximity of body to wire

        If the body and the wire are not in contact, whether an object touched the wire and body, acting as a conductor

    D.   Voltage and amperage

    E.   Clothing on subject, particularly at point of contact

    F.   Condition of subject

        1. Whether perspiring

        2. Physical condition

    G.   Rigor mortis

—30—

EXPLOSION

SYNOPSIS

Death as a result of explosion is usually accidental in nature, but may be caused by suicide or homicide (Fig. 66)

In these cases, samples of the debris and the powder, together with a detailed description and photographs of the scene, are necessary to determine the cause, and the exact point of the explosion.

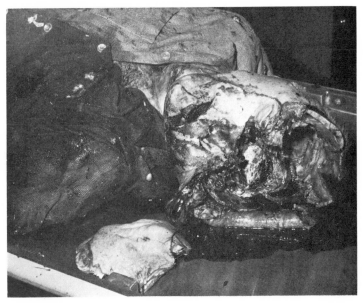

FIG. 66. Explosive injury to head.

Because of the very nature of an explosion, the victim is usually disfigured to such an extent that identification is very difficult; therefore, for purposes of identification itself and for purposes of establishment of a corpus delicti, careful search should be made for any dismembered parts of the victim or for pieces of his clothing or jewelry that can help in this identification.

In addition to the search, the investigator should thoroughly question all possible witnesses who, firstly, saw any subjects in or about the premises immediately preceding the explosion, and, secondly, any witnesses who heard the explosion, in order to determine the number of such explosions, the description of the sounds of same, the approximate location from which these sounds came, and the appearance of the flying debris and smoke that followed the explosion.

No debris, powder, dust or anything in the immediate vicinity should be disturbed until an explosive expert is summoned.

EXPLOSIVES

I. General

Upon discovering a bomb, suspected bomb or any other explosive material, a must is to call a trained expert to dismantle, remove or detonate it

II. Experts

A. Chemical companies

B. U. S. Army

C. Local F.B.I.

III. Positive steps to be taken before arrival of expert

A. Clear danger area

B. Obtain services of expert

C. Avoid moving any article or object which may be connected with the explosive or act as a trigger mechanism

D. Guard boundaries of danger area

E. Shut off power, gas and fuel lines leading into area

F. Remove flammable materials from surrounding areas

G. Notify local fire departments and rescue squads

H. Notify medical aid to stand by

I. Place sand bags, mattresses, etc., to protect against flying fragments

J. Have fire extinguishers handy

K. Secure portable x-ray equipment, on stand-by

Note: Do NOT convey any known explosives or bombs to headquarters or laboratory before consulting the expert and obtaining his specific recommendations

—31—

GUNSHOT WOUNDS

SYNOPSIS

A slug will normally take a straight path through a body and, if the speed and momentum is great enough and no objects such as bones struck, will pass completely through the body.

If the velocity of the bullet is not great, or if it strikes bones or certain tissues, its path may become uneven and bent. If the bullet strikes a soft part of the body (e.g., the brain) it can produce an explosive aspect, and the bullet will break into several parts.

Because of the different types of powder, amount of powder in the cartridge and other factors, it is very difficult to determine the exact range of a shot. Here again only tests by experts by comparison shots, microscopic examination of the powder residue and chemical analysis of the powder and metal can determine with any accuracy approximate distances and material used (Fig. 67).

Contact wounds often do not reveal powder burns on the surface, the same being under the epidermis and visible only when the wound is examined internally.

Powder residue and burns are likewise sometimes deposited on the clothes of the victim and are important in determining trajectory of the bullet and position of the subject when the gun was fired; for example, a powder burn on the shoulder and sleeve with an entrance wound near the neck could indicate the fact that the arm of the deceased was raised when the gun was fired. For this

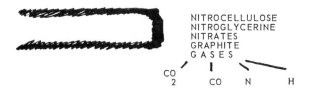

AS BULLET LEAVES MUZZLE, ACCOMPANIED

BY GAS, FLAME, SMOKE AND BURNED AND

UNBURNED GRAINS OF POWDER.

FIG. 67. Substances leaving muzzle of gun with bullet.

reason, removing the clothing of the deceased or unnecessarily rolling or crumpling same may lead to confusion in later examination. This is also true with bloodstains on the person and on the clothing; these stains, together with the burns, should never be touched or disturbed in any manner or to any degree.

In case of suicide, the gun is usually held by the victim against or very close to his skin. Usually a right handed person will shoot himself from the right side, but this is not always the case, in that a person may use his thumb to set off the trigger rather than holding the gun as one normally does to fire at a foreign object. The hands of the deceased will sometimes offer important clues in this respect, showing either marks caused by the recoil of the gun or blood from the spattering of the wound.

Great care should be taken to distinguish facts at the scene to help indicate whether a death by gunshot wound is as a result of murder, accident or suicide, and no conclusion should be drawn until the subject is closely examined by a pathologist. (Forms 12-15—Identification of Guns) (Form 16—Firearm Distance Chart) (Form 24—Gunshot Report) (Forms 48 and 49—Firearms and Powder Residue Identification Tests)

GUNSHOT WOUNDS

I. When death is apparently due to a gunshot wound, it is necessary for the investigating officer to determine

    A. Whether death is due to the gunshot wound or to an injury inflicted by some other instrument

       (Stab wounds often resemble gunshot wounds)

    B. If by a gunshot wound, from what distance the firearm was discharged

    C. The direction from which the shots were fired

    D. The position of the body when hit

    E. Whether it was accident, suicide or murder

II. Investigation

    A. Scene

       1. Diagram, measure and photograph weapons, slugs, cartridge cases and richochet marks, being careful not to move, mar or contaminate any clues

       2. Use extreme care in the handling of the weapon

          a. Do not place pencil or other instrument into barrel in removing

          b. Use precaution in not adding or removing fingerprints

          c. Consider every gun loaded

       3. Inspection of weapon

          a. To determine

            (1) Make

        (2) Model

        (3) Serial number

        (4) Whether loaded

        (5) Number of discharged bullets contained therein, and

        (6) Number of loaded bullets contained therein

   4. Position of weapon in relation to body

   5. Angle of weapon in relation to body

   6. Ejected cartridge cases and their location

   7. Buried slugs

B. Body

   1. Number of wounds

   2. Location of wounds

   3. Appearance of wounds (Fig. 68)

   4. Appearance of areas adjacent to the wounds

   5. Determination of entrance and/or exit wounds

   6. Apparent course of the slug

   7. Whether the course was altered

   8. Whether the slug struck an object before striking the body

   9. Whether projectile passed through clothing before entering the body

  10. Whether projectile struck a bone in its course through the body, thereby

     a. Altering its course

       OR

     b. Splintering the bone, thereby creating additional exit wounds or apparent trajectories

  11. Whether there is more than one projectile in any one of the wounds

F. Firing—as projectile leaves muzzle, it is accompanied by
  1. Flame from burning powder
  2. Unburned particles of powder and carbon
  3. Soot
  4. Grease
  5. Particles from barrel
  6. Oil from barrel
  7. Gases from explosion
    a. Nitro-cellulose
    b. Nitro-glycerine
    c. Nitrites
    d. Nitrates
    e. Gases graphite
    f. CO_2, CO, N, H
    (Fig. 67)

IV. Wounds
  A. Bullet
    1. Has velocity (speed)
    AND
    2. Rotation
    3. Slowing up on contact with the skin or any other object
    4. Producing an indentation
    5. Being accompanied by flame, burnt and unburnt particles of carbon, gases, etcetera
    AND
    6. Containing lubrication, grime, dirt, etcetera
  B. Entry wound
    1. May be black from lubrication, grime, flame, etc.

2. Usually smaller than the exit wound, depending on
   a. Ammunition
   b. Distance from which weapon was fired AND
   c. Clothing, etcetera, covering the subject

Note: Relationship between the size of the entry wound to the exit wound equals the distance of the muzzle from the body surface

3. Distance (See Fig. 69)
   a. Contact
      (1) Tight
          (a) Abraded ring from contact
          (b) Pattern of muzzle on skin
      (2) Loose
          (a) Burning
          (b) Smudging
          (c) Some tattooing
      (3) General
          (a) Gases expand in skin and subcutaneous tissues, creating
              1) Larger entry wound
              2) Jagged, everted edges
              3) Severe injuries to deeper tissues by explosion
              4) Blackened skin, even in deeper tissues

Note: Gas escaping cannot penetrate body and attempts to force its way out, creating tears and jagged areas; however, gas may penetrate the surface where there are soft tissues

Note: In contact wounds hair can be singed, and a mark of the barrel from the recoil can sometimes be clearly seen

Note: Angle of weapon can sometimes be seen by the imprint of the powder on the skin.

  b. 2″ to 6″—near contact
    (1) Smudging—black and solid
      Residue of powder and flame
    (2) Tattooing
      Residue of individual flakes of powder
    (3) Flame from gun might burn skin

  c. Close range—6″ to 18″
    (1) Entrance wound is smaller than exit wound
    (2) Oil from projectile might be present
    (3) Smudging
    (4) Tattooing (light)
    (5) Powder embedded in skin

  d. Intermediate—18″ to 24″ (hand gun)
           Up to 30″ (Rifle)
    (1) No burning
    (2) No smudging
    (3) Powder—may be present

  e. Distant
    Small particles are absent

  f. General
    (1) Type of entrance wound may vary with the type of gun
    (2) Powder in a bullet does not usually burn all at one time (gelatin content)

      (3) To check distance, investigator
         should
         (a) Fire same gun
         (b) Using same type of bullet
      (4) With high velocity weapons
         (a) A splash-back may be creat-
            ed, tearing the tissues and
            causing an entrance wound
            to resemble an exit wound

C. Exit wound (Fig. 70)
   1. Usually larger than entrance wound

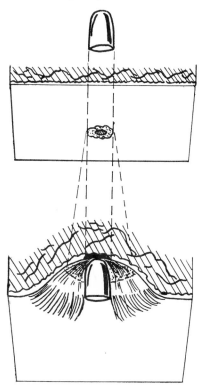

Fig. 70. Entrance and exit of bullet.

2. Frequently irregular in shape
3. More blood than entrance wound leakage
4. Everted, round or oval—no powder burns
5. Larger where solid organ or bone is hit near exit— (Secondary missiles—several exit wounds)

V. Effect on body (Fig. 71 and Fig. 72)
    A. Depends on energy transmitted

$$\text{Energy} = \frac{M \times V_2}{2}$$

    B. Shape of projectile
        Blunt, rounded, etcetera
    C. Stability of projectile

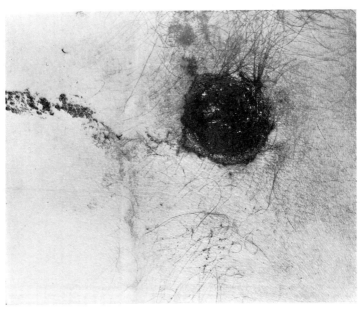

Fig. 71. Entrance hole.

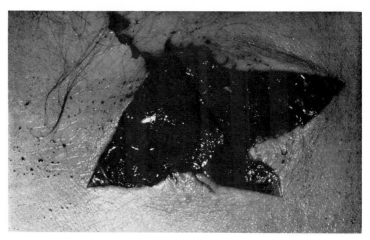

FIG. 72. Exit hole.

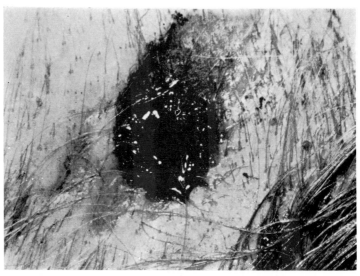

FIG. 73. Entrance hole, showing contact wound when gun held
at slight angle.

D. Resistance of tissues of body to entrance of projectile

Note: When projectile strikes body, called "terminal ballistics" (Fig. 73).

VI. Shotgun
   A. General (Fig. 74)
      1. Rate of spread
         a. 1 inch per yard from muzzle plus 1
      2. Lethal potential depends on
         a. Number of shot
         b. Velocity
         c. Penetrating shot
         d. Amount of choke in the gun (potential is increased by the choke)

   Note: Choke is the narrowing of the barrel

Note: Range of average shotgun approximately 50 yards

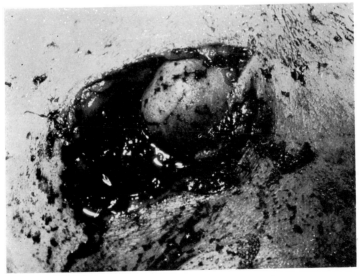

FIG. 74. Entrance wound from shotgun (contact).

B. Investigation
1. Up to 1 yard—single wound, with much burning, blackening and tattooing (Fig. 75)

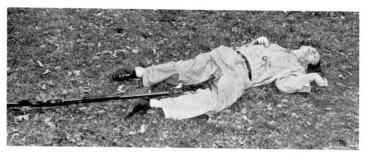

Fig. 75. Powder burn pattern shown on clothing (loose contact).

2. 1 to 3 yards—larger wound; burning and blackening are not present, but slight tattooing occurs
3. Over 3 yards, tattooing disappears and shot disperses
4. Wadding (compressed paper or padding to separate powder from shot or to keep shot from falling out of the cartridge)
    a. Seldom travels beyond 40 to 50 feet
    b. After a distance of approximately 5 feet, wadding begins to drop before the primary wound
    c. Will mark body up to about 10 feet
C. Spread in inches

	5 yds	10 yds	15 yds	20 yds	30 yds	40 yds
Cylinder	8	20	26	30	45	60
Half choke	5	12	16	20	32	45
Full choke	3	9	12	15	25	40

VII.   Collection, preservation and shipping
  A.   Firearms
      1. Record place where found by photo-
          graphs, notes and diagram
      2. Remove gun with several fingers on the
          side of the trigger guard

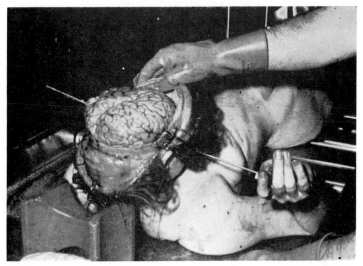

Fig. 76. The above indicates proper method to photograph trajectory of bullet, especially in determination of a self-inflicted
wound.

      3. Never submit a loaded gun to laboratory
          unless it is personally delivered
          a. Unload
          b. Submit clips and cartridges separately
      4. Do not clean the gun in any way
      5. Take care not to destroy any fingerprints
      6. Note position of gun in relation to other
          objects

7. Note make, model and serial number of gun
8. Note condition of gun
   a. Smell
   b. Smoke
   c. Loaded or fired cartridges
   d. Misfires
   e. Temperature of barrel
   f. Position of safety mechanism
   g. Position of hammer or cocking mechanism

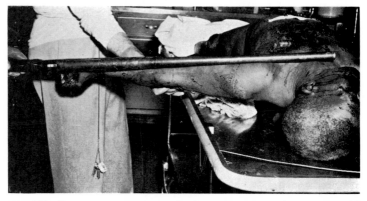

Fig. 77. Determination as to whether or not wound was or could have been self inflicted.

9. Identify gun by marking same (Small mark on barrel)
10. Place in suitable container
    a. Place in cotton, paper, etcetera
    b. Pack rigidly in box
    c. Wrap securely
    d. Obtain receipt when turned over to someone else

11. For comparison, also obtain for evidence all ammunition, shells and bullets

B. Cartridges
  1. DO NOT mark cartridges, cases or clips
  2. DO NOT clean or wipe off before packing (may contain blood, hair or fibers)
  3. Place in cotton or soft paper
  4. Place in a box
  5. Seal the box
  6. Initial same

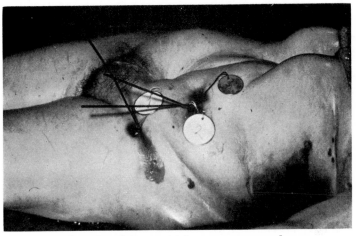

Fig. 78. Probes identifying multiple entrance wounds.

7. For comparison, also obtain all other ammunition and suspected firearms
8. Before removing be certain to photograph, sketch and measure location of all cartridges and cartridge cases, in relation to and on what angle from body and guns

Note: Never remove the cartridge or slug with any instrument, thus protecting same from being marred or disfigured

—32—

INDUSTRIAL DEATHS

An industrial death is one that occurs during and in the course of employment, as a result of other than natural causes.

A coroner's inquest into these types of death has more legal significance than in any other type, in that: (1) employers must be notified of the hearing; (2) lawyers are allowed to interrogate witnesses; and (3) the transcript is admissible at a later compensation hearing as evidence.

Investigation should be conducted in the usual manner, except that the investigator should also determine actual employment of the victim, his employer, the type of work that he was assigned to do, the type of work that he was doing, and the manner in which the death occurred. Although a death during and in the course of the employment creates an industrial death, for purposes of paying compensation, it is still important to discover whether there was civil or criminal negligence on the part of any other person or persons.

Oftentimes a death may occur in the course of employment which is, in effect, a natural death, and cannot, as such, be considered in this category.

—33—

INFANTICIDE
SYNOPSIS

Infanticide is the killing of an infant after birth. Even though an infant may not have breathed, the deed may still be infanticide if the subject was capable of living.

Usual methods of committing infanticide are by strangling the child by the umbilical cord, suffocation, drowning or merely exposure by leaving in a hidden place.

Finding the wrongdoer is extremely difficult in this type of crime, in that pregnancy is usually hidden and the parents almost impossible to find.

How the umbilical cord was cut might determine if there was help of a professional. Preservation of the afterbirth can lead to identity of the mother and the father by determining the blood type of the child from the child itself, the blood type of the mother from the afterbirth, and the blood type of the father by cross comparison of the other.

This is also possible by preserving the articles in which the baby was wrapped for examination of blood and prints. Cloth or bags might give a clue as to environment and neighborhood of the wrongdoer, or of the business places which he or she frequents.

Hair or other stains on child or wrapping are also important clues.

(Form 46—Fetus Age Determination Chart)

INFANTICIDE

I. Definition

The act of killing an infant soon after birth

II. Pre-requisites
   A. Must be shown that infant could have lived under normal care
   B. Accepted criterion of normal formation and gestation period is usually at least 20 weeks
   C. Must be shown that the baby was born alive
   D. Cause of death must be established

III. Usual methods of infanticides
   A. Drowning
   B. Dropping in toilet commodes
   C. Smothering
   D. Throwing from heights

IV. Body usually found in
   A. Garbage or refuse containers
   B. Sewer disposal plants
   C. Roadsides
   D. Alleyways

V. Determination of age
   A. General
      1. Stillbirth — 28 weeks gestation or over, born dead
      2. Fetus — under 28 weeks
   B. Measurements
      1. Over 28 weeks of gestation
         a. At least 14″ long
         b. At least 2½ pounds in weight

   2. Fetus
      a. Less than 14″ in length
      b. Two and one-half pounds, or less
  Note: A fetus can be subject to infanticide
      or murder
   3. Scale of measurements
      a. First five months of gestation
        (1) Measure from crown of head to
            underside of its buttocks (rump)
        (2) Measurements should be in centi-
            meters (2½ centimeters equal 1″)
        (3) Square root of above equals the
            age of fetus in lunar months
      b. Last five months
        (1) Measure in inches from heel to
            top of head
        (2) Measurements, when divided by
            two, will give the approximate
            age in lunar months
      c. Weight
        (1) Five lunar months—approximate-
            ly one pound
        (2) An increase of one pound each
            month until 36 weeks
        (3) Then weight of approximately
            five pounds
        (4) Last four weeks—approximately
            one-half pound each week
VI. Investigation of possible infanticides (Fig. 79)
   A. Umbilical cord
      1. Cut (?)
      2. Forceps used (?)
      3. Post-natal dressing (?)

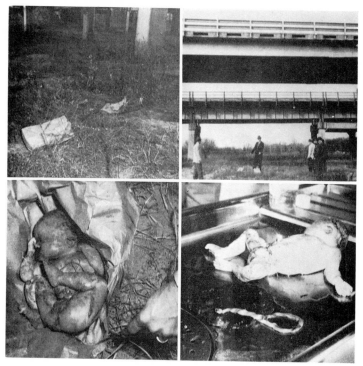

FIG. 79. Infanticide. Series of pictures showing location where child was found, place from where it was thrown, bag in which it was wrapped, umbilical cord and string tying same, and afterbirth.

From blood in the baby and blood on the bag and afterbirth, the blood types of the baby, mother and father were determined. Tying of cord and string showed the work of an amateur. Child was killed firstly by suffocation and later thrown off the bridge from a passing auto.

        4. Professional tying of umbilical cord
        5. Note drying (to show separate existence)
  B.   Evidence
        1. Wrappings

2. After-birth (placenta)
   to determine
3. Fingerprints
   AND
4. Blood typing

Note: By determining the blood type of the infant and, either from the after-birth (placenta) or wrappings, the blood type of the mother, the blood type of the father may also be determined

5. Autopsy essential
   a. To determine possible cause of death
   b. To determine if infant could have lived under natural circumstances
   c. To determine possibility of separate existence
      (1) Air in lungs
      (2) Air in the stomach
      (3) Drying of the cord
      (4) Food in the stomach to determine if it had been fed
      (5) Bruises
      (6) Presence of bacteria in the blood stream

      Note: A stillborn baby with no separate existence has not breathed and is, therefore, sterile and contains no bacteria

Note: A stillborn infant is not subject to postmortem putrefaction

—34—

LIGHTNING

I. Nature
   A. Millions of volts and thousands of amperes from clouds where generated and then transferred to the earth where they are neutralized
   B. Main flash usually gives off subsidiary flashes; Area may be as much as one hundred feet in diameter

II. Injuries
   A. Similar to those received from electrical current
   B. Metallic objects on body may be magnetized or fused
   C. Release of heat and "secondary flash" may
      1. Tear clothing
      2. Throw off clothing
      3. Eject metal objects

III. Investigation
   A. If there was an electrical storm at the relevant time
   B. Scene—other signs of lightning (burnt grass, effect on tree, etc.)
   C. Fused metal objects on or near body
   D. Magnetism of some metal objects
   E. Examination of subject himself for
      1. Signs of electrocution
         AND/OR
      2. Signs of burning

—35—

DEATH BY POISON
SYNOPSIS

Determining whether a person died as a result of natural illness or as a result of poisoning is one of the most difficult types of investigation both for the officer and for the medical expert. Symptoms of different kinds of poisonings include vomiting, convulsions, coma, dilatation or contraction of pupil, paralysis, changes of respiration, delirium, cyanosis and the like; however, unfortunately, for the investigator and for the medical expert, these symptoms are also present in various types of normal deaths.

The first prerequisite in this complicated field is suspicion. An investigating officer should at all times be on the alert for possible poisoning and, wherever there is the slightest suspicion of same, should conduct a full and complete investigation at the scene; any laxity in this investigation can very conceivably hinder and hamper the pathologist and medical technologist in the discovery and proof of the presence of poison.

In cases where there is a suspected poisoning, a complete and very thorough search should be made of the premises where the deceased is found. A very important factor to remember is that in practically every case the preliminary determination that the death was due to poisoning can only be made by investigation and examination at the scene, and, only at that time can it usually be decided that, if it was poisoning, whether or not same was as a result of murder, suicide or accident. An autopsy by the pathologist at a later time and examination of stomach contents or the like by the medical technologist can only determine the amount of poison used and the quantity; oftentimes, in the failure by the officer to discover the actual poison used, the medical technologist might conceivably be stymied as to the discovery of the particular type of poisoning. The presence of any one poison is so difficult to ascertain that it may be undetected unless the examiner has some idea as to the type of poison for which he is looking.

Care—extreme care—should be taken to preserve any form of evidence discovered.

Interrogation of witnesses can provide information which may be very important to the toxicologist; and this type of information should include the food and drink that the person has had within the past 24 hours, the last time he ate or drank anything, the symptoms and complaints of the person, the first appearance of poisoning and the symptoms of poisoning, his reaction—whether he vomited, urinated, went into convulsions or into delirium—and this interrogation should also provide information as to whether the subject was in good health prior to this time, and all other information that might have any bearing at all in such a matter. Also ascertain whether or not any other persons ate the same foods or drank the same liquids as the deceased, and, if so, who they were and what they ate or drank; a check should then be made to determine whether any of these persons have suffered any ill effects.

Whenever there is any suspicion of poisoning, it is suggested that the officer conduct his criminal investigation, but that he permits nothing to be disturbed in the house or at the scene itself, and that experts be summoned so that no possible clue to the establishment of the proof of poisoning is disturbed or overlooked.

The overlooking of a clue may very conceivably result in the failure on the part of the pathologist, medical technologist or toxicologist to discover the presence of the poison or the type of poison; some poisons can likewise disappear or be destroyed through embalming and putrefaction; only some poisons do not disappear with time. Arsenic can be detected for many, many years after death, and carbon monoxide can be detected for a certain period of time after death; on the other hand, such poisons as cyanide, hypnotics and the like disappear in varying periods of time anywhere from a few months to eighteen months or two years.

It must be observed that poisoning is one of the easiest ways for a person to commit murder and get away with it, firstly, because of difficulty in detecting the same; and, secondly, because of the fact that the person who administers the poison is usually a close friend or a member of the family, and that the unsuspecting officer is often misled by not knowing the circumstances which led to this murder. It is also not uncommon for one to commit suicide by reason of poison and yet fail to leave a suicide note of any type; and, in the person's neatness in replacing the bottle from which he took the poison to the medicine cabinet, fail to leave the important clues which would indicate the fact that he did take his own life.

Thusly, in any suspicious death or in any death unattended by a doctor, it is recommended that a complete investigation be made, and that even where the death is apparently a natural one, that the officer make every effort to locate every type of medication or possible poison that may be on the premises and to keep the same as possible evidence.

(Form 23—Poison Report) (Form 45—Poison Chart)

POISON

I. Definition

An agent, which when introduced into an organism in a greater than safe quantity, may chemically produce an injurious or deadly effect

II. General

A. Cause of death
1. Shock
2. Pneumonia
3. Perforation of stomach
4. Late complications
5. Direct action on nervous system

B. External appearance depends on
1. The poison itself
2. Concentration of poison
3. Volume of poison
4. Period of time poison is in contact with soft tissue before death and after death
5. Smell

C. Specific poisons
1. Narcotic
a. Ultra short acting
b. Short acting
c. Intermediate acting
d. Long acting
e. Mixed
2. Aspirin
a. Fatal dosage for adult—500 gr. or 100 5 gr. tablets
b. Death may be delayed over 12 hours

3. Alkaloids (opium, etc.)
   Like other narcotic deaths
4. Cyanide
   a. Smells like bitter almonds
   b. Bright pink color
   c. Corrosive on lips
   d. Froth coming from mouth
5. Insecticides
   a. Excessive thirst
   b. Vomiting
   c. Contraction of pupils
   d. Odor
   e. Immediate onset of rigor mortis after death
6. Carbon monoxide
   a. Colorless, odorless
   b. Combines with hemoglobin in blood
   c. Replaces oxygen
   d. Red cells (which carry CO_2) unable to carry sufficient CO_2 to support vital organs
   e. Appearance
      (1) Cherry red color
      (2) Vomiting
      (3) Fluid from nose and mouth
      (4) Bladder and bowels may empty
   Note: Delayed death may occur and carbon monoxide may be practically absent from system
   f. Sources
      (1) Car exhaust (7% carbon monoxide)
      (2) Coal gas, etc.
7. Chronic drug addiction

        8. Natural gas—lack of oxygen in air
           a. Death by suffocation
      Note: It takes less oxygen to keep person alive than fire going
      Note: Oxygen comprises 20% of air
      Note: 1½ quarts of air in respiratory system

III. Investigation of scene (Fig. 80)
    A. Medicine bottles
    B. Tubes
    C. Hypodermic needles
    D. Pills, capsules and the like
    E. All empty medicine containers
    F. Used utensils, cups, glasses, etcetera
    G. Particles of food
    H. Soiled linen
   Note: Oftentimes in both murder and suicide attempts will be made to conceal the act by either hiding the containers or placing them in their usual sites (medicine cabinets and the like)

IV. Deceased
    A. Evidence of convulsion (note unusual features that the subject might have that could have been caused by convulsion)
    B. Vomiting or excretion
    C. Peculiar odors
    D. Presence of stains or powders on the victim or his clothing
    E. Intense cyanosis (caused by depression of the respiratory system)
    F. Petechial hemorrhage of skin (pin-like spots)
    G. Mucus about the mouth
    H. Burn marks on the lips

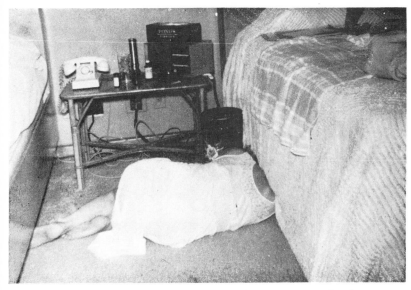

Fig. 80. Death due to self ingested barbiturates. Note bottles on table with caps tightly screwed on and in apparently original position. Other illustration shows total medication, barbiturates, tranquilizers and poisons found in drawers, medicine cabinets and closets throughout the house. Fatal dosage actually came from Tuinal found in medicine cabinet and not from either of the two bottles on the table. Points out necessity of taking-in everything as possible evidence.

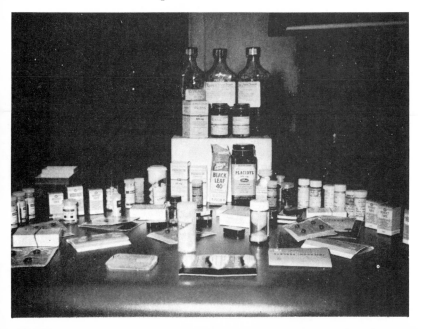

Note: X-rays may determine the presence of lead poisoning

Note: Metallic poisons, such as arsenic and mercury, may be determined from skeleton many years after death

V. Interrogation of witnesses
   A. Obtain information important to toxicologist
      1. Food and drink that the deceased has had in the past 24 hours
      2. Last time he ate or drank anything
      3. The first appearance of poisoning
         a. Whether deceased vomited
         b. Urinated
         c. Went into convulsions or delirium, etcetera
   B. Whether deceased was in good health prior to this time
   C. Whether any other persons ate the same food as the deceased (if they did, then these persons should be checked to determine whether they have suffered any ill effects)
   D. Any prior threats or attempts of suicide
   E. Where poisons and medicine are usually kept
   F. From where poisons or medicines were obtained
   G. Physician, if any, attending the subject
      1. To determine moods of subject
      2. To determine medications prescribed
      3. To determine date prescribed and amount prescribed
      4. To determine physical ailments of deceased

VI. Evidence
    A.   From scene
        1. All medicine bottles, tubes, needles, pills and the like
        2. All empty or partially empty poison or medicine containers
        3. All utensils apparently used for recent eating or drinking by the deceased
        4. Samples of food that the deceased may have recently eaten
        5. Samples of excretion, saliva, vomit, urine, blood, etcetera
        6. Stained sheets or clothing, etcetera
        7. Any object that may have been used to administer the poison

VII. Evidence from body (Fig. 81)
    A.   Poisons such as arsenic may be detected for many years after death
    B.   Carbon monoxide may be detected for a certain period after death
    C.   Other poisons such as cyanide, hypnotics and the like, disappear in varying periods anywhere from a few months to 18 months
    D.   Embalming makes the discovery of many poisons and medications extremely difficult
    E.   Autopsy to be done before the body is embalmed
        1. Stomach
        2. Liver
        3. Kidneys
        4. Brain
        5. Lungs
        6. Heart

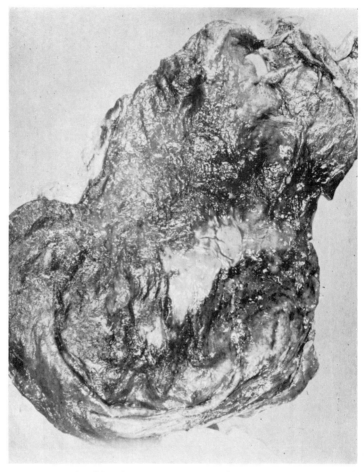

FIG. 81. Hydrochloride acid poisoning showing hole in stomach and loss of lining.

7. Spleen
8. Blood
9. In case of arsenic poisoning, nails and hair of victim

Note: Each medication should be submitted in a separate clean glass container, without the adding of any preservatives (preservatives do not necessarily destroy the poisons or medications but may make them more difficult to detect)

VIII. Collection, preservation and shipping of evidence
    A.   Food specimens
        1. If already in a suitable container (such as a fruit jar) close and seal same
        2. If not in a food container, place in a clean glass container
        3. Seal tightly
        4. Label
    B.   Vomitus, urine, etcetera
        1. Place in a clean glass jar
        2. Seal with a tight fitting lid
        3. Label
    C.   Chemicals (solids, powders, tablets, capsules, etc.)
        1. Obtain all to no more than one pound
        2. Place in clean individual wrappers or dry glass containers
        3. Submit with all other solids suspected of being identical or suspected of having been used for comparison purposes
    D.   Chemicals (liquids, such as oil, gasoline, medication, waters, etc.)
        1. Obtain all to no more than one quart
        2. Place in dry sterile glass containers with tight lids
        3. Submit together with all liquids believed to be identical or which could have been used for comparison purposes

Note: The determination of poison contained in a deceased should *NOT* be limited to merely examining stomach contents; the presence of a poison in the blood stream and in the brain is a pre-requisite for proof of the effect of this poison on that individual

IX. General classification of poisons
  A. Gases (e.g., carbon monoxide)
  B. Anesthetics (e.g., chloroform)
  C. Corrosives (e.g., cyanide)
    1. Strong mineral acids
    2. Strong alkaloids
  D. Metallic (arsenic)
  E. Organic (e.g., opium)
    1. Alkaloids
    2. Non-alkaloids
  F. Food poisonings

—36—

SEXUAL ATTACK

I. Investigation
    A. Photograph for minute detail
        1. Scene
        2. Subject
    B. Hair
        1. Pubic and genital hairs important
        2. Do not cut hair, but pull same out by the roots
    C. Stains
        1. Semen
        2. Blood
    D. Clothing fibers, etc.
    E. Fingernail scrapings
   Note: Test for virginity of subject
II. Accused
    A. Samples of hair
    B. Samples of blood
    C. Sample of semen
        To be obtained from clothing, and more particularly, underclothing of accused
III. Seminal stains
    A. Clothing of victim and suspect, or defendant
    B. Manner of obtaining
        1. Cover stain with clean piece of paper
        2. Fold so as not to disturb
        3. Pack each piece individually
        4. If wet, dry or handle carefully, so as not to disturb or spread stain

C. Also obtain
    1. All clothes or material in immediate area
    2. Smears from the victim (to be taken by Doctor) (Fig. 82)

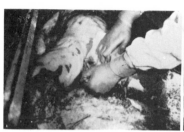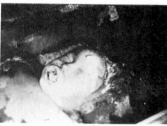

Fig. 82. Drowning victim and subsequent examination for possible sexual attack.

IV. Common sex crimes
    A. Masochism
        Sexual perversion by inflicting pain on oneself or having pain inflicted on him
    B. Sadism
        Sexual pleasure by inflicting pain on someone else
    C. Fetishism
        Sexual pleasure by using female clothing or seeing same on the body of the victim
    D. Pederasty
        Homosexual pleasure by penetrating the anus of another male (usually inflicted on a child)
    E. Rape
        Forcible entry without consent of female
    Note: Investigation of these deaths will usually show many signs of external maltreatment on wounds and many indications of a struggle
    Note: Sex violators are often repeaters, and investigation should be conducted with this theory in in mind

—37—

STABBING AND CUT WOUNDS
SYNOPSIS

Knife wounds are generally classified as wounds by cutting, stabbing or slashing.

Most important factors are the shape, length, sharpness and characteristics of the knife, place of the wound or wounds and manner of entry. Holes and tears in the clothing are very important in reconstructing the scene and should not be disturbed except under close direction of the pathologist, who can compare and align these holes and tears with the wounds themselves.

The investigator should not be misled by either the total depth of a stab wound or the exact length of a knife, in that the murder knife itself might conceivably be shorter than the total length of the stab wound or the stab wound much deeper than the length of the knife blade. This apparent inconsistency is caused by pressure against the skin, forcing the skin and bones to "give a little."

Another important factor is whether and how an injury caused death, and in the case of multiple wounds which one was the fatal wound; careful investigation and a thoroughly and carefully performed autopsy are necessary to reach definite and correct conclusions.

STABBING AND CUT WOUNDS

I. General

Death from stabbing and cut wounds is seldom accidental, but rather almost always

    A. Homicidal

       or

    B. Suicidal

II. Incised wounds

    A. General

       1. Inflicted by an instrument with a sharp cutting edge

       2. At times stab wound and gunshot wound may look alike

       3. A fall on a sharp object, such as ice or hard floor, may create a laceration which might resemble knife wounds

    B. Appearance

       1. Normally straight

          BUT

       2. May be irregular where the penetration is an area of lax tissue

       3. Margins of wound cleanly cut

       4. No bruising of the wound areas

       5. Tissues cleanly divided

       6. Tends to gape, creating more bleeding than other types of wounds

    C. Self inflicted

       1. Usually in front of a mirror

       2. Suspicion of blood usually on the mirror itself

3. Wounds multiple and parallel, and usually in one area (usually neck, wrist or ankles)

4. Hesitation marks noticeable (superficial cuts an inch or so long at the point of origin, indicating that the subject first tried out the edge of the instrument before he made the final gash)

5. Usually commences from left to right with a right handed victim (from right to left with a left handed victim)

6. When on neck, wound will pass slightly downward and then straight across the neck

7. Clothing is usually not cut, but is removed from area that wound is inflicted

8. When death follows cutting of throat, knife or other cutting instrument will oftentimes be found clenched in hand (cadaveric spasm)

D. Homicidal

1. No premeditation or hesitation marks exhibited

2. Wound on neck will usually be on the side or back of the neck

3. Defense wounds—when a person is defending himself, he will instinctively throw up his arm to protect his face, and gashes or cuts will be found across his arm, wrist or hands (Fig. 83)

4. Clothing is cut

5. If victim had an opportunity to defend himself, blood stains would be scattered over a considerable area

III. Stab wounds

A. General
Usually homicidal

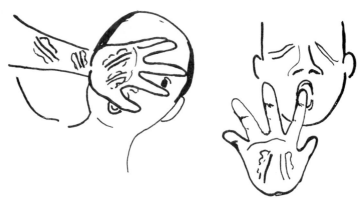

Fig. 83. Illustrates typical locations of defense wounds, depending on position of hands of victim in attempting to ward off blows.

    B. Nature and extent of wounds depends on
        1. Type of weapon used (Fig. 84)
            a. Area
            b. Shape
            c. Length
            d. Sharpness
            e. One or two edged
        2. Manner used
        3. Part of body affected
        4. Depth of stabbing
        5. Position of body
        6. Stature and physical condition of assailant
    C. Blood distribution
        1. Small artery
            Spurts with drops of blood as they strike surface
        2. Large artery
            Bleeding rapid and profuse
        3. Vein
            Flow or gush out

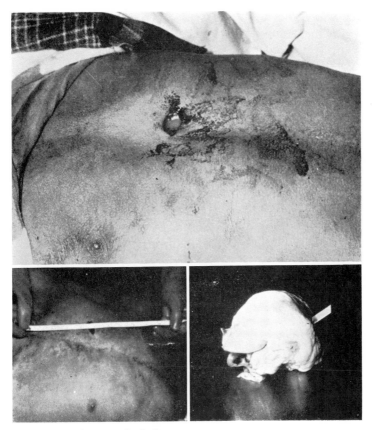

Fig. 84. Knife wound of chest.
Examination to determine type of knife, width, angle of blow and depth of penetration.

IV. Chop wounds
  A. General
     Usually homicidal
  B. Usually inflicted on exposed parts of the body
  C. Force usually in a downward or partially downward direction

    D. Note

       Usually inflicted by hatchet, ax, claw part of hammer, etcetera

V. Weapons

    A. Examine them for

      1. Fingerprints

      2. Foreign material

        a. Fiber from clothing

        b. Dust

        c. Hair

        d. Skin

        e. Blood stains

      Note: Blood will not always adhere to a fast moving, smooth, metallic object; thusly, it is possible for a knife which was a murder weapon to be devoid of blood (the same applies to an ice-pick or like weapon)

    B. Preserving evidence

      1. Place at the bottom of a strong cardboard carton lined with clean white paper

      2. Fasten to bottom of carton

      3. Place clean paper on top of weapon

      4. Close and seal with gummed paper

      5. Protect suspect weapon from possible contamination by other fingerprints, dust, fibers, liquids or the like

    Note: Where multiple wounds are apparent, extreme care should be used in not spreading stains or removing clothing, so that every tear in the clothing may be correlated with the wound beneath same

    Note: Fingernail clippings should be taken to determine possibility of a struggle and for possible identification of the assailant

—38—

EFFECTS OF ALCOHOL
SYNOPSIS

When one consumes alcoholic beverages through the mouth, the alcohol is swallowed and is then passed through the esophagus into the stomach; it is then absorbed through the stomach walls, most of it passing into the small intestine and into the blood stream. The rate of this absorption varies, depending upon the physical condition of the person and upon certain other factors, but generally speaking most of the alcohol consumed is absorbed within approximately one hour after consumption. The alcohol that is absorbed in the blood stream is then pumped throughout the whole body; since alcohol has a characteristic of following and finding water and since there is an element of water in all parts of the body, then that alcohol necessarily distributes itself to all the parts of the body and is stored in those parts in proportion to the amount of water located there.

Once the alcohol reaches the various parts of the body, especially the area of the brain and nervous centers, it adversely affects and partially paralyzes the thinking and nerve apparatus of the human being. The effect that this alcohol has upon the brain and upon the nervous system depends to a great extent upon the physical condition of the person, the amount of alcohol he has consumed, his absorption rate, his tolerance, and the elimination of alcohol from his body.

The concentration of alcohol in the brain and nervous center as brought to the brain by the blood first impairs the judgment of a person; then it causes a muscular incoordination, followed by stupor and unconsciousness, and possibly, after a certain period of abnormally large consumption, death.

It is possible with reliable accuracy to test this concentration of alcohol in the human being. Actually, when an alcohol test is given, it, in effect, measures the difference between the amount of alcohol absorbed, as hereinbefore set forth, and the amount that is passed off from the body. Alcohol is usually always absorbed through the mouth. Contrariwise, it is usually passed off through one of the following media: oxidation (burning off), urination, exhaling through the lungs and bleeding.

The standard method of testing the alcoholic content in an individual is from the blood, urine or breath; all of these methods are basically founded upon the fact that the alcohol becomes equally distributed in the fluids of the body. The fundamental measure of alcohol is the percentage of that alcohol in the circulating blood and, whether the tests are taken from the urine or from the breath, saliva or the blood itself, the net result is determined by the concentration of alcohol in that blood.

Because of the reluctance of some people to be literally stuck with a needle, and because of the absolute medical and scientific requirements of a person who would conduct such a test, the more used and practical method of testing for alcoholic concentration is the breath, and the principal machines used for such tests are the drunkometer, the intoximeter and the alcometer. These various machines range in size and price, but they have two main things in common: firstly, that the person taking such a test should have experience and expert background; and, secondly, that any of these tests merely measure the alcohol influence upon the person by means of measuring the percentage of alcohol in the circulating blood.

The concentration of alcohol in the blood is measured by tenths of a per cent. When this concentration is less than 0.05 grams per cent alcoholic content, it may be presumed that the person is sober and that his thinking apparatus and reflexes have not been affected or impaired. It is not uncommon to find anywhere from 0.01 grams per cent to 0.03 grams per cent in a person, even though that person has not consumed any alcoholic beverages; this is based upon the normal alcohol concentration in all human beings.

However, when the concentration exceeds 0.05 grams per cent, but is less than 0.15 grams per cent, a question arises as to whether or not that person is under the influence of intoxicating liquor; some persons may be under that influence and some may not, although it is more than probable that when the concentration is beyond 0.10 grams per cent that person's reflexes and thinking ability will be hampered .

When that concentration exceeds 0.15 grams per cent, regardless of the person's physical condition, his absorption rate, tolerance, previous experience in drinking, or any other factor, there seems to be no doubt at all either in scientific or legal circles that that person is definitely under the influence of intoxicating liquor, and that his ability to act and to reason has been impaired.

From 0.15 grams per cent alcoholic content in the blood to 0.22 grams per cent, the person finds himself in a state of excitement; from approximately 0.20 grams per cent to approximately 0.35 grams per cent the person is in a confused state, and from approximately 0.25 grams per cent to 0.45 grams per cent the person finds himself in a semiconscious condition or in a stupor; over 0.35 grams per cent the person is completely unconscious, and at 0.45 grams per cent to 0.55 grams per cent may find himself on the verge of death.

An alcohol test, in addition to determining the percentage of alcoholic content that the person has at the time of the test, can also permit an estimation, with reasonable accuracy, of the amount of alcohol concentration of that person at the time of an accident or of an arrest at a known period of time before that test was taken—assuming that that person had nothing to drink since the time of that accident or the arrest, and also assuming that he had nothing to drink for approximately one hour before the arrest.

It should be the policy of a coroner's office to test the presence and percentage of alcohol concentration in all persons who survive for less than twelve hours before a death by violence; it is important that this test be done and be obtained before any embalming procedure is instituted, which procedure may destroy and make meaningless any subsequent alcoholic test.

Examination of the deceased for alcohol is an important factor in reconstructing the manner of death, the cause of death, and the motives or reasons that precipitated the occurrences leading to same.

Alcohol from a deceased should be taken with blood from the heart, stomach contents, brain, urine in the bladder, liver, kidneys and/or spinal fluids.

In order to obtain an accurate analysis, consideration is given to the amount of hours a person lived after he last consumed the alcohol and the amount of hours he lived after he suffered his injury, in order to determine the exact alcoholic content in that person at the time of the injury; in addition, some consideration is given to the length of time the person is dead, in that, through a putrefaction process, which is similar to a fermentation, a person might very conceivably build up from a 0.02 grams per cent alcoholic content to a 0.08 grams per cent alcoholic content; and, by the same token, persons who have a very considerable amount of alcohol in them at the time of their death, may lose some of this alcohol during this putrefaction process.

A study by the Coroner's Office in St. Louis County has revealed that, generally speaking, 20% of all deaths investigated are violent. This study further reveals that approximately 50% of all violent deaths are either directly or indirectly caused by intoxication of one of the principals involved. This percentage varies in the type of death; for example, alcohol plays a part in over 50% of all fatal automobile collisions and murders, but, contrariwise, contributes only approximately 5% to such accidents as falls, electrocutions, etc.

Regardless of how complete and how thorough an investigation is made by a police officer of an automobile collision and fatality, it is unfortunately very improbable and almost impossible that that officer, with the evidence that he is able to secure under the limitations that the law imposes upon him, will be able to obtain a conviction against the wrongdoer. There is nothing more discouraging, nor is there a greater let-down to a law enforcement official, than when he sees a person who he knows is guilty of taking another person's life and of taking that life while violating the law go free with little or no punishment, and than when he sees this miscarriage of justice repeating itself time and time again with no movement on the part of his fellow men to rectify this unfortunate situation.

It is the duty of the coroner, when he determines that there is an underlying cause of an unusually large number of deaths in his community and when he determines the means with which these deaths can be greatly reduced, to inform the public officials and the people of that large number of deaths and of the possibility of that reduction. The uniform chemical test for intoxication act is such a means; in effect, it sets forth the following:

(1) An implied consent of the driver of a motor vehicle to submit to chemical testing to determine alcoholic content of the blood;

(2) Persons qualified to administer these tests;

(3) Consent of person incapable of refusal not withdrawn by the fact that he is dead, unconscious or the like;

(4) Revocation of privilege to drive motor vehicle upon the refusal of the arrested person to submit to chemical testing;

(5) Administrative hearing on request of the person whose privilege to drive has been revoked or denied to determine whether that revocation or denial was properly done;

(6) Judicial review of same;

(7) Interpretation of the chemical test (basically the same as hereinbefore set forth in this chapter);

(8) Proof of refusal to take the test admissible in any civil or criminal action; and

(9) The provision of this act would not limit the introduction of other competent evidence bearing upon the question of whether the person was under the influence of intoxicating liquor or was intoxicated.

The investigator, in order to make his thorough investigation and to protect the innocent and convict the guilty, is permitted certain latitudes and rights, including examination of personal property, automobile, clothing, wounds, physical features and the like; an alcohol test is one more step on that long road of humanity and civilization that permits complete criminal investigation and opens the door to his final goal, conviction of the guilty and protection of the innocent.

(Form 28—Alcohol Report Form)

ALCOHOLIC INTOXICATION

I. Measuring standards (Fig. 85)
    A.   .05 gms % — .15 gms % — under influence
    B.   .15 gms % — .22 gms % — excitement state
                             — intoxicated
    C.   .20 gms % — .35 gms % — confused state
    D.   .25 gms % — .45 gms % — stupor

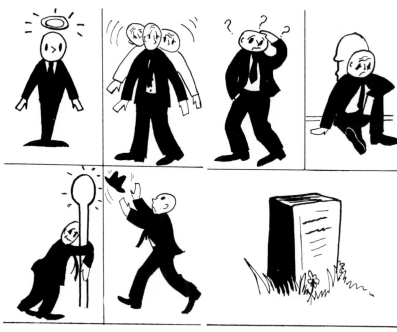

F<small>IG</small>. 85. Tests for intoxication are important in determining background and reasons for every type of violent death. Tests taken on all violent deaths in the St. Louis County Coroner's office over a five-year period indicate that intoxication is directly and/or indirectly involved in more than 50 per cent of ALL violent deaths.

E. .35 gms % and over — unconscious

F. .45 gms % — .55 gms % — on verge of death

II. Amount of alcohol to affect person

    A. .04 gms %

        1. 2 bottles of beer

          OR

        2. 2 ounces of 100 proof whiskey

          FOR

        3. 150 pound person

    B. .15 gms %

        1. 6 bottles of beer

          OR

        2. 6 ounces of 100 proof whiskey

          FOR

        3. 150 pound person

    C. Liquor absorbed approximately one hour after consumption, depending on

        1. Make-up and condition of the drinker

        2. Food in the stomach

        3. Tolerance

    D. Approximately 1 ounce of whiskey or one bottle of beer dissipated in approximately 3 hours

III. Process

    A. Absorbed through the mouth to esophagus

    B. Then to large intestine

    C. Then to small intestine and liver

    D. Then into blood stream, finding water in blood stream

    E. Then to rest of body, including brain and nervous system

IV. Passed off through

    A. Oxidation

    B. Kidneys (urine)

    C. Exhaling through lungs

    D. Bleeding

    E. Perspiring or sweating

  V. Manner of tests

    A. Blood

    B. Urine

    C. Breath

 VI. Examination of living subjects (Fig. 86)

    A. Pre-requisites

      1. Consent of subject

      2. Consciousness of subject

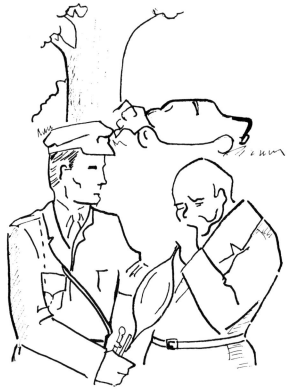

FIG. 86. Intoximeter (balloon) test.

B. Additional observations of subject
    1. Demeanor
    2. Smell
    3. Reflexes
    4. Memory
    5. Co-ordination
    6. General appearance
C. Necessary exclusions to prove intoxication
    1. Injury
    2. Shock
    3. Natural diseases or sicknesses
    4. Medication or dope
  Note: Alcoholic content may be increased after death through putrefaction (fermentation) from 0.02 gms % to 0.08 gms %
  Note: Sometimes may be reduced through same process
  Note: Alcohol test should be made of all deceased persons dying as a result of possible violence, as additional information to explain circumstances surrounding death

—39—

SUICIDES

Suicide ranks second only to deaths by automobile collisions as a leader in number of violent deaths. It occurs more frequently than murder and is usually more easily predicted, in that, generally speaking, before one attempts suicide, he has either previously attempted to take his own life or has threatened to take it, or has written a suicidal note that he is about to take his own life. More than 17,000 people a year, and approximately once every minute, somebody in the United States either kills himself or attempts to kill himself. Aiding a man in committing suicide in practically every state is a crime; suicide itself is a crime, and, in most states, if the court or law enforcement officials so desire, persons who attempt to commit suicide could be punished for attempting to commit a crime. Religiously speaking, suicide is a law against every type of church in existence, and was first recognized as a law against the church in 452 A.D. In the Common Law, a person who committed suicide would forfeit the estate by so doing. Proportionately, many more "whites" commit suicide than negroes. The general reasons for committing suicide are numerous, but basically speaking, the more "popular" reasons seem to be as follows:

(1) General depression caused by pain, loss of mind, ill health, divorce and the such;
(2) Sex maladjustment;
(3) Homosexual relations;
(4) Thought of gaining immortality;

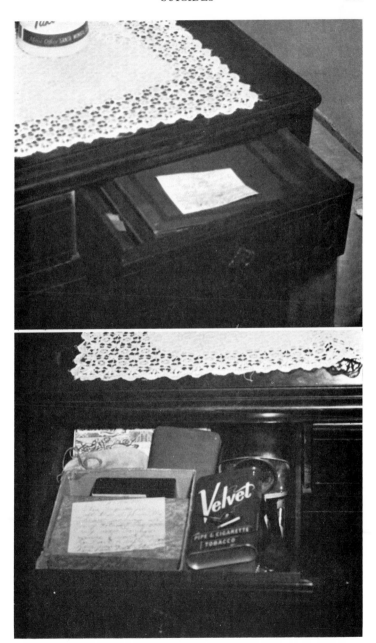

Fig. 87. Suicide notes. Note they are hidden in drawers, and how victim wrote two such notes and put them in separate drawers.

(5) Escape of unbearable situations;

(6) Desire to kill;

(7) Desire to be killed;

(8) Loss of love;

(9) Loss of self-esteem;

(10) Revenge (a guilt complex for those alive);

(11) A loss of usefulness in life.

It is important for the investigating officer to know the above facts, in that, in his investigation, by determining the health, physical condition, and the background of the individual, he might be helped in establishing whether the death was actually caused by suicide, and also determine why suicide, if such is the case, was committed.

Sometimes an officer is called upon to investigate deaths where apparently one of the persons took the other's life and then his own.

It behooves the officer to determine in this case what an autopsy or pathological examination may not be able to find, to-wit:

(1) Which one inflicted the mortal wound on the other?

(2) Who died first?

(3) Was there a struggle?

(4) Was there any evidence of killing in self defense?

(5) Was there a suicide pact?

(6) Why?

Position of the bodies, location of weapons, ownership of same, notes, and marks on the hands are vital pieces of information in this type of investigation (Fig. 87).

—40—

MASS CASUALTIES

The public, generally, and officials in particular, including Coroners themselves, are prone to minimize the role that a Coroner's Office can and should play in the event a disaster strikes its area.

In recognizing the possibility of having death spread its dark hands over a large section of his community, the Coroner must necessarily be prepared to assume the responsibility that will be his at that time. He must further realize that where disaster strikes and help is needed, even though no deaths have been reported, it behooves him to utilize his trained personnel and his specialized equipment to supplement the work of police, fire, civil defense, medical and health agencies.

The Coroner must recognize the fact that upon his shoulders rests a great responsibility, and that unless his department is properly trained and organized to meet that responsibility, havoc, uncertainty, fear, crime and disease could be inflicted upon his fellow citizens.

I

CATASTROPHIC DISASTER

The least occurring, but most difficult, disaster with which the Coroner would have to deal is the one of major or catastrophic proportions. Every community is potentially subject to such a disaster, which could conceivably almost totally destroy that area and the people therein. Such an unfortunate occurrence could be the result of an enemy attack, a tornado, cyclone, fire, flooding or the like. Once he recognizes the fact that these dangers do exist, and that deaths might result in a very large magnitude, he must overcome his reticence and prepare for same.

Firstly, the Coroner should make arrangements with the proper reporting agency (whether it be civil defense or police) to notify him. Forthwith, he should notify several designated personnel in his office, and they, in turn, should be prepared to contact a like number—all of this being done in a chain-like motion until the whole staff is properly put into operation. To properly so operate the Coroner's Office should be divided into the following categories.

1. Administration.
2. The collecting and transporting of the dead.
3. Morgue facilities.
4. Autopsy and pathological examination.
5. Photographing, fingerprinting and other identification facilities.
6. Embalming and disposition of the bodies by burial or cremation, where necessary.
7. Health services.

8. Storing and protection of personal property found on the bodies.

9. Definite records of the deceased.

10. Religious services.

11. Releases to the family, press, and public, generally.

Upon receiving notification of a major disaster, and after making the proper 'phone calls, the Coroner, a stenographer, at least one deputy and a transportation and burial expert, should proceed to the civil defense control center, from where they will direct operations of the mortuary service.

Other deputies will be distributed in Coroner radio cars and at the sector morgues and assembly areas, where they will direct transportation and other predesignated assignments.

The teams that are assigned to the devastated areas should be responsible for the proper tagging of all bodies, along with the recording of all pertinent information on these tags. Personal effects should be kept with the body until it is delivered to the morgue and removed with the clothing under proper medical and investigative supervision. In loading of bodies, extreme care should be taken not to intermingle any personal effects or clothing. Wherever possible, mortuary bags or wraps should be used.

Upon the arrival of the trucks at the staging area or morgue, the following procedure should be used:

1. Mortuary wraps should be removed and death confirmed by a qualified medical practitioner.

2. Identification teams should record all basic data, personal effects and basic description data, including the taking of photographs and fingerprinting when possible.

3. The bodies should be so tagged or marked, so that upon removal of these identifying factors the per-

sonal effects can be readily traced to that particular body, or vice versa.

4. Steps should then be taken to preserve the personal effects on the body.

5. Close examination of the body should be made by the Coroner's Pathologist, with help from a medical technologist and x-ray technicians, to attempt to definitely establish the exact cause of death.

6. Arrangements for burial should then be made, utilizing charts and markers to indicate location of all interments.

7. Clergy should be used for observation of proper religious rites.

Understanding, of course, that every public office is dependent upon budgetary limitations, it is suggested that, within proper limits, the Coroner's Office should have at its disposal adequate mortuary wraps, grave markers, identification tags, portable x-ray equipment, and a mobile laboratory and autopsy room. In addition thereto, the Coroner's Office should have on call qualified personnel who could be available to supplement the regular employees in the event of these emergencies.

The Coroner, in planning such an operation, must take into consideration that it is his duty not only to establish the cause of death and the identification of the deceased, but also to protect the property of the deceased, to keep posted the press, the family and other interested persons, and to determine the presence of any sickness, diseases or foreign matters that might be contagious or dangerous to the community as a whole.

In this particular category, more than in any other one discussed herein, it is imperative that the Coroner put his staff through mock exercises, so that in the event this contingency ever arises, each member will be prepared to assume the responsibility assigned to him without further instruction or supervision.

The personnel of this staff should at least include, but not be restricted to, the following: the Coroner, deputy coroners, pathologists, funeral director, morgue attendants, transportation advisor, chaplain, x-ray technician, medical technologist, photographer, fingerprint identification expert, and secretary. Each of these personnel should be made a leader over his or her particular unit, and every person within that Coroner's Office should be advised that no bodies will be released, nor any information divulged to anyone, except by way of and under the direction of the Coroner himself.

II

LOCALIZED DISASTER

A localized disaster differs from and cannot be handled in the same manner as a catastrophic disaster discussed above. In that such a disaster is usually confined to a particular area, the Coroner's work must necessarily originate at the scene.

After the pending dangers are eliminated by the fire and police departments, and after the area is cleared of the untrained personnel, the Coroner's Office should then, in conjunction with the fire department and police department, take charge of the scene.

Firstly, the area should be roped off to keep the scene from being over-run by sight-seers, hysterical people and souvenir hunters, and to preserve that scene in as close to its original state as is possible; secondly, guards should be posted to preserve and protect the property located thereon; and finally, investigators from the Coroner's Office and other interested departments should be designated to conduct an "on the spot" interrogation and investigation.

The Coroner, himself, should be accompanied by a stenographer, a photographer, a pathologist, and at least one investigator.

He must keep in mind that no general plan can be set forth here or at any one particular time to govern every situation; it is necessary that a common and orderly set of procedures be agreed upon and followed at the scene by and between all the departments involved, each department cooperating with and supplementing the work of the other department.

It is important to remember that every bit of information available at the scene may be essential in uncovering clues that might be indispensable in helping determine the identity of the body and the causes of the fatality; with this in mind, care should be taken not to rush the removal of any of the bodies or any of the evidence until this investigation is concluded to the satisfaction of all departments.

Where a large number of deaths has been caused by an explosion, all evidence should be utilized to the fullest to attempt to determine its force and extent, the effect of this explosion not only on the bodies but on equipment and personal property, and whether it was in one main body or if a group of smaller explosions may have occurred at one spot or in a number of spots. The force of the explosion, parts of bodies and personal possessions within certain distances must be carefully studied to piece together the unknown and to aid in the collection of parts of human beings and in the careful assembling, marking and identifying of these parts as belonging to one person or to another. As explosions are often accompanied with fire, this close and careful investigation could and must reveal whether the death and damages were caused through the explosion, burning, inhaling of carbon monoxide or other poisonous gases.

To the same extent this is true in an airplane crash. The scattering of possessions and bodies must be carefully analyzed, both for identification purpose and also to determine whether the cause of death was from fire, from gas, from direct contact upon the crashing of the airplane, or from the body being thrown from that plane; likewise, the determining of whether these bodies or properties were scattered around the area of crash or in a direct line with the crash may lead to the conclusion that the plane may have exploded before it hit the ground, that it hit the ground head-on, or that it skimmed along the ground and exploded and burst into flames as it was moving. Again, any such information is necessary in establishing the cause of the death and the cause of the crash and disaster, and in making such an investigation any small particle of the airplane that might be carelessly moved or removed may seriously hamper this investigation. A careful and detailed description of all personal property and all baggage and suitcases, and especially all clothing and types of clothing and materials and laundry marks, must be meticulously recorded and preserved as evidence.

Detailed drawings, stenographic services and portable recording outfits should be used to provide complete and detailed reports to be expanded upon and studied at some later time.

Another type of localized disaster is a fire. Where such a fire occurs at a public dance or in a theatre or bowling alley, unusually careful attention should be given to the type of clothing and the type and amount of jewelry worn by the apparently unidentifiable individual and to his or her physical description.

No attempt at identification should be made at the scene, but all bodies, together with all information, should be immediately removed to the morgue and identification or attempts to identify made at that place. In the event of a fire in a hospital, nursing home or school of any type, however, extreme care should be exercised not to remove the bodies until such time that the principal, superintendent or person in charge, in conjunction with the aid crew, helps them reconstruct, on paper, a description of the building, so that it might be determined in what part of that building the certain individuals were found; then, as these bodies are located, they should immediately be tagged as to the portion of the building in which they were discovered, and as to whether or not any part of that building was beneath them or on top of them, or whether one person was lying by himself or with a group of other people or below or above another person. Then as these bodies are removed, one at a time, a careful notation should be attached to the body as to the location from whence it was taken, the position in which it was found, the particles of building or materials that surrounded it or were underneath or near the body, the clothing and jewelry and personal possession located above, beneath or near the body, and at the same time this body should be numbered and that number should be placed in a proper position on the sketch of the building previously drawn. Again, no attempt should be made to identify the body at that particular time, but the corpse should be removed from the scene in an ambulance (one at a time), and with extreme care being taken in the loading and unloading of these burnt beings, so that when further study is made at the morgue none of the valuable evidence that was gathered at the scene is lost, confused or misplaced.

In all manners of disaster, where a body and its facial features are destroyed, process of elimination can be an important element in the identification of an individual, and oftentimes one name can be established principally by the elimination of other known names; frequently there is confusion and hysteria in attempting to determine the number of individuals involved, and this can hamper the identification of all persons who might have been in the disaster. In these cases, especially where bodies are severed, it is important that each part be properly identified and a note of the exact site of recovery attached to that part; if it can be determined at the scene that any of these parts belong together, they should be put in one group and wrapped together, properly marked, so that they will not be accidentally separated at a later time. The exact location of these parts and the position that they take to the other parts of any one body may be of the utmost importance in establishing the number of dead, and by one process or another, either by definite identification or by elimination, in identifying all of the dead. By the same token, whenever it is determined that there are any articles which may belong to any one body, these articles should be kept with the body, and wrapped with the body in such a way that they cannot be lost.

As these bodies are removed from the scene, a careful supervision should be maintained by a member of the Coroner's Office, and he should precede the delivery of these bodies to the morgue, so that a definite and complete explanation can be given to those in charge at the morgue as to the relevant facts that were observed at the scene.

Assuming that the number of dead from any one localized disaster such as discussed above would conceivably be less than one hundred, the usual County Morgue and its surrounding rooms and corridors can be properly equipped to receive, store and handle the bodies recovered from such disaster, and to accommodate the investigative and administrative units.

This area would be under the exclusive jurisdiction of the Coroner, his deputies and assistants, and should be closely supervised and controlled, so that the area set forth by his Office for certain personnel will not be used by any unauthorized persons.

Waiting rooms should be provided for immediate relatives of possible disaster victims. Another room should be provided for the purpose of interviews and investigations. A stenographer or recording units should be made available in each of these rooms. Three rooms should be made available as viewing rooms, each of these rooms to be used, respectively, as follows: one for males, one for females and one for children. Another room should be made available for property, although no such property should be distributed unless it is authorized both by the police department and the Coroner's Office. An area should be set aside for use of clergy and another one for use of the press. The autopsy room should be kept clear and that, together with x-ray equipment, should be placed under the complete supervision of the pathologists. Arrangements should be made for the taking of fingerprints and photographs of the victims.

The personnel should consist of the Coroner, two deputy coroners, two stenographers, photographers, fingerprint experts, pathologists, x-ray technician, dentist, chaplains, investigators in charge of public relations, a homicide expert, a pharmacist, a tailor and morgue attendants.

Upon reaching the morgue, one at a time, each body should be separately numbered, and a duplicate record made—one copy of which should be kept in the record room and one copy with the body itself.

This record should state all the particulars of the discovery of the body, the time it arrived at the morgue, and as personal identifications are made they should be checked out and marked on the record. These elements of identification are as follows:

1. Apparent sex.
2. Approximate age.
3. Measurements of body.
4. Height.
5. Weight.

6. Scars.
7. Type and color of hair.
8. Type and color of eyes.
9. Glasses, if any.
10. Nose.
11. Ears.
12. Mouth.
13. Shape of head.
14. Complexion.
15. Type of beard.
16. Teeth (last longest)
    a. Missing
    b. False
    c. Fillings
    d. Defects
17. Physical condition
    a. Apparent illness or operations.
18. Fingerprints.
19. Blood type.
20. Type of hands.
21. Social status.
22. Environment.
23. Occupation.
24. Jewelry
    a. On what hand or fingers.
25. Clothes
    a. Size
    b. Material
    c. Color
    d. Value
    e. Laundry marks
    f. Weaving or tears.
(See Forms 29, 32 and 33)

In the case of a localized disaster, the proper recording of facts, the use of these facts and the release of information obtained from same to the public, and proper censoring when necessary, may have a great effect upon the family of victims involved, upon the community in which the disaster occurs and, in a majority of cases, upon all communities throughout the entire country. Therefore, before any such releases are made or information divulged, a public relation committee, composed of the delegates from the various departments involved in the handling and investigation of the disaster, should assemble and discuss the matter in detail and determine between them who shall release what information. It is recommended that these departments consist of no less than the police department, the fire department, the medical staff and the Coroner's Office.

The absolute necessity of close supervision in such disasters may more readily be seen in the fact that the lack of same may permit premature, misleading and false information which may be alarming or inaccurate, and may —simply in the fact that it is premature—allow the criminal or the guilty to conceal their identity and/or their wrong-doing, and may create unnecessary hysteria. Pressure by relatives, political subdivisions, the press and the public generally must be ignored, and such a release must wait until all the relevant information is completely digested and understood by all departments concerned, and until those departments are certain that the information they give out is accurate and correct.

In the case of many localized disasters, the remains of a human being disassembled and the parts thereof scattered may cause confusion in determining the exact number of bodies or fatalities involved in that disaster; in addition thereto, the finding of parts of flesh or pieces of bones may not necessarily reveal that these belonged to human beings, in that in their damaged or burnt state the bones or flesh may appear to be human and have all human characteristics but in reality be animal or fowl.

A certain and definite identification of a possible disaster victim is admittedly needed for moral and religious reasons, but it is also necessary for all legal intents and purposes, and the absolute and positive establishing of the death of a person certainly is necessary to establish that death for legal intents and purposes. Although the bereaved family may be chagrined and irked at the delay and seemingly slow process of the Coroner's Office, such certainty will in the long run prevent delays and inconveniences in the collection of insurance policies by the beneficiaries, and in the clearing of titles of the person's property and real estate, and perhaps will allow a later remarriage by the surviving spouse. Unless this definite identification is made, it is conceivable that that person may still be alive, or that he will be presumed to be alive by law, and that the surviving family or spouse may be forced to wait a period of time until that person will be presumed to be legally dead under the laws.

Even though a body may be identified beyond any reasonable doubt, the removal of such body shall not be authorized by the Coroner until it is completely and fully examined by the Coroner's pathologist, to determine accurately and definitely the cause of that particular death. It is possible and probable that, although a disaster of any particular type transpired, the deaths were caused by more than one reason; for example, in any disaster caused by an airplane crash, explosion or fire, it is found that deaths are caused from trauma by impact in falling, from burning, from carbon monoxide poisoning and sometimes from natural causes whereby a person with a weak heart or other natural illnesses may be affected through fear or shock or over-exertion.

Also necessary before any body can be released is the taking of photographs of each of these bodies for viewing at a later time by any person who is doubtful as to the identification of any disposed of body, the taking of finger-prints, so that same may be checked by the proper agencies for definite identification, and for the taking of x-rays, so that the body may be examined and permanent records made of his bone structures and other unseen factors that might help in definite identification; the purpose of these is to again establish certainty and to erase doubt.

During the identification process in the morgue itself and rooms adjacent thereto, and the dispersal of the dead, Coroner's investigators shall be assigned, along with investigators from the various departments involved and selected experts in the particular field involved in the disaster, to assemble evidence, take pictures, interview witnesses and gather whatever information they deem is necessary in order to determine the possible causes of this disaster, the responsibility of individual or individuals involved and all relevant information concerning the disaster itself; this investigative committee should make a permanent record of all of its findings and should form a conclusion as to whether or not prosecution of any individual should be instituted by the state, and also recommend any possible steps that might be taken in the future by the public generally or by any public official in this or any other community to prevent or minimize any such future like disaster. At the completion of this investigation, the Coroner, together with the investigative committee and the heads of the various departments, shall meet in order to determine the scope of an inquest or inquiry, and to determine who shall be summoned; a jury should be selected for such inquests, composed of citizens of the county who are experts in that particular field and, as such, will be capable of arriving at an intelligent decision concerning the cause or causes of deaths involved, together with centralization of responsibility and obligation, and recommendations for the elimination or minimizing of such future disasters.

At this inquest, all witnesses to the disaster shall be permitted and requested to testify, and all the material gathered in the identification and investigations prior to the inquest shall be made a part of the record.

In addition thereto, all departments shall be requested to make written criticisms and recommendations of the procedures of investigations of these disasters, so that, in addition to all the information as outlined above, lessons can be learned and transmitted to other disaster units throughout the country, and a more efficient method and manner of handling, investigating and reporting any such future disasters may be effectuated.

Only by supreme and voluntary cooperation, and by systematic and intelligent handling of a localized disaster by officials of various departments involved, can every bit of information that is possible be learned from that disaster; otherwise, time, money, manpower, and most important of all, lives, are literally wasted.

III

RESCUE

It is recognized that immediate control of any disaster lies strictly within the hands of the police and fire departments and medical and health agencies; it is their duty to supervise the rescue of the living and injured, and to see that they are properly cared for and identified; it is further their duty to effectuate a reconciliation between them and their loved ones as soon as possible. However, the Coroner must also lend whatever manpower and equipment is at his disposal to insure that these facilities are not wasted, to the detriment of the wounded and needy. He should keep in mind the fact that every Coroner's Office contains a certain number of trained personnel, including those qualified in medical, technological and investigative work. Therefore, upon a report of any major disaster, even if no deaths have been recorded but where injuries and damages are prevalent, the Coroner's Office should be notified by local civil defense or police officials, and his trained staff should be ready to supplement other investigative and rescue units. His medical personnel should be utilized in the rendering of first aid to the wounded, and his trained personnel should be used in conjunction with local civil defense and police officials in the removal and identification of the wounded, the notification to the relatives and the press, and the preservation of property and possessions. During this phase of operation, the Coroner's Office is, of course, under the direction of the proper departments.

MASS CASUALTIES

I. At scene (Fig. 88)
  A. Rope off and guard area
  B. Permit only trained personnel in area
  C. Do *NOT* hurry
  D. Work slowly and methodically
    1. Study type of disaster
      a. To determine location of bodies or parts of bodies

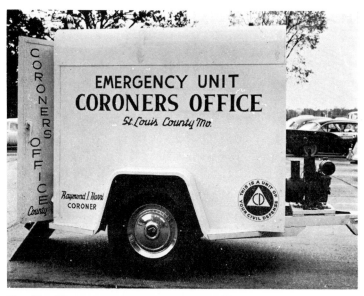

FIG. 88. Emergency or investigative trailer.
Contents: generator; extra lighting; shovels; spades; cameras; recorder; cots; blankets; roping-off, portable investigative, evidence gathering and first aid equipment, etcetera.

          b. To look for evidence

      2. Outline procedure
         AND
         Assign tasks

      3. Search carefully
          a. Wrap and mark remains separately
          b. Note place where found
          c. Note names of recovery crews
          d. Preserve other evidence
          e. Draw map and take pictures

II. Conveying remains to morgue
    A. Supervise removal
    B. Do *not* allow removal until records are complete
    C. Do *not* allow removal until morgue facilities are ready

III. At morgue
    A. Do not admit outsiders until everything is ready
    B. Assign casualty numbers
    C. Have all forms available for description and labeling
    D. Follow morgue procedures

IV. Relatives
        Do *NOT* permit identification until information sheets are filled out and signed by them regarding persons they wish to identify

−41−

EXHUMATION
SYNOPSIS

Exhumation is the disinterring or digging up of a body, once buried. Although the disinterring of a body is a very rare procedure, it is sometimes necessary for one of the 3 principal following reasons: (1) when the body has been improperly or illegally buried to conceal a death or a crime; (2) where the cause of death as certified to in the death certificate is questioned; and (3) when the identity of the buried person must be either verified or disproved.

It is desirable, but practically and financially unfeasible, to autopsy deaths of all types—violent, presumably natural, where no doctor is in attendance, and "naturals," where an attending physician is willing and does sign the death certificate. The unfeasibility of universal autopsies of all deaths emanates from the financial, religious and practical restrictions existing in almost every given jurisdiction.

In addition thereto, so-called complete autopsies sometimes fail to reveal an exact cause of death, particularly where the administration of certain poisons, narcotics or tranquilizers is not suspected and is unknown to the investigator, the pathologist and the medical technologist at the time of the autopsy. This weakness is even further exaggerated by the current medical inability to trace and determine the presence of a multitude of tranquilizers presently in use.

Thusly, it can be seen that it sometimes becomes necessary to exhume a body after it has been placed in its final resting ground. The legal procedure necessary to authorize exhuming of a body differs in the various jurisdictions, and any officer or Coroner should first consult his local District or Prosecuting Attorney before proceeding to do same, so that there is an assurance that such exhuming is legal and proper, thereby protecting the officer or Coroner from a possible civil law suit by the relatives of the deceased, and thereby further allowing any discoveries resulting therefrom to be introduced in evidence in court. Regardless of the local laws, a written consent from the proper relatives is desired, but not necessary, before the exhumation.

The officer or Coroner must remember that the exhuming of a body is not only to discover a previously unknown factor regarding the death, but also to be able to utilize the said discoveries for purposes of investigation and final trial.

EXHUMING OF A BODY

I. At the grave
   A. Persons present
      1. Coroner
      2. Police
      3. Family
      4. Cemetery Official
      5. Grave digger
   B. First identification
      1. Cemetery Official
      2. Grave digger who filled the grave originally
      3. Person who made and/or erected the grave marker
   C. Opening of grave:
      1. A sample of dirt on the surface of the grave, together with samples from several other sections of the cemetery
      2. A sample of soil approximately 1 foot above the coffin
      3. Coffin top cleaned and identified
      4. Photograph of the coffin in the grave
      5. Samples of dirt from all 4 sides of the coffin
   D. After the coffin is removed
      1. Photograph of the coffin
      2. Samples of soil from the terrain beneath the coffin
      3. Samples of water in the grave aperture, if any water is present

II. At the morgue
   A. Persons present
      1. Coroner

      2. Police
      3. Family
      4. Undertaker
      5. Pathologist
  B. Procedure in removal of body
      1. Lid removed and body identified by undertaker and family
      2. Samples of shroud and clothing
      3. Samples of fluid or water in the coffin
      4. If coffin is of wooden construction, samples of wood
      5. Removal of the body
  C. Examination of body
      1. Pictures of the body
      2. Samples taken of fungus or other growth on the body
      3. Autopsy
         a. Samples of internal organs, especially the hair, nails, skin, muscles, bone, blood and urine
         b. Where there is suspicion of poisoning, the above samples should be carefully handled and should not be diluted by placing them in containers containing other chemicals

III. Legal procedure
  A. Through Court order, as specified by the laws of the respective jurisdictions, or
  B. By consent of legal, qualified next of kin

—42—

GUIDE TO WORDS

Abortion: Uterus empties itself prematurely; criminal abortion is a willful production of a miscarriage of a woman who is pregnant, whether by administering drugs, or using instruments or by any other means, but only when not being necessary to save her life.

Abrasion: Wearing away of the skin in small shreds by friction.

Accident: An unforseen occurrence, especially one of an injurious character.

Acid: Any compound of electronegative element.

Adipocere: Peculiar waxy substance formed during the decomposition of animal bodies, and seen especially in human bodies buried in moist places. It consists principally of insoluble salts of fatty acids—called also "grave-wax," (soap-like appearance).

Acute: Sharp.

Afterbirth: The mass cast from the uterus after the birth of a child (placenta).

Alcoholism: The effect of excessive indulgence in intoxicating liquors.

Amnesia: Lack or loss of memory, especially in remembering past experiences.

Anatomy: Study of the structure of the human body.

Anemia: Insufficient oxygen-carrying capacity of the blood.

Anesthetics: A group of drugs capable of producing either localized or general loss of sensation. Example: (1) chloroform—heavy, colorless liquid with a characteristic odor and taste; (2) ether—colorless, volatile liquid with penetrating odor.

Aneurysm: A sac formed by the dilation of the walls of an artery or of a vein and filled with blood.

Angina: Spasmodic pain.

Ante mortem: Before death.

Antidote: A remedy for counteracting a poison.

Antitoxin: A substance found in the blood serum and in other body fluids which is specifically antagonistic to some particular toxin.

Anoxia: Oxygen cannot gain access to blood stream; lack of oxygen either locally or generally.

Anus: The distal end and outlet of the alimentary canal.

Aorta: The great trunk artery which carries blood from the heart to be distributed by branch arteries through the body.

Arrest: The seizing of a person and detaining him.

Arsenic: A medicinal and poisonous element; it is a brittle, lustrous, graying solid, with a garlicky odor.

Arson: The intentional and illegal burning of a dwelling house or out-house—usually a felony. There are different degrees of arson, depending on type of dwelling burned.

Artery: Any one of the vessels through which the blood passes from the heart to the various parts of the body.

Asphyxia: Suffocation.

Aspiration of vomitus: Breathing or drawing in vomitus into the respiratory tract, blocking same.

Assault: An unlawful attempt with force of violence to do bodily hurt to another.

Asylum: An institution for the support and care of the helpless and deprived classes, such as the insane and the blind .

Autopsy: The internal examination of a body after death.

Barbituate (or barbiturate): A salt of barbituric acid.

Cadaveric spasm: Stiffening and rigidity of a single group of muscles occurring immediately after death.

Canine: Of, pertaining to, or like a dog.

Carbon monoxide (C O): A colorless and odorless gas.

Carbon dioxide (C O$_2$): A heavy, colorless gas.

Cardio: A combining form denoting relationship to the heart.

Cardiovascular: Pertaining to the heart and blood vessels.

Cartilage: The gristle or white elastic substance attached to articular bone surface and forming certain parts of the skeleton.

Castration: Removal of the gonads (primary sex organs).

Cavity: A hollow place or space.

Cerebral: Pertaining to the cerebrum, which is the main portion of the brain occupying the upper part of the cranium.

Cervical: Pertaining to the neck.

Chronic: Sickness of long duration.

Circulation: Movement in a regular course; as the circulation of blood.

Cirrhosis: A disease of the liver, marked by progressive destruction of liver cells.

Coagulate: To cause or to become clotted.

Colon: That part of the large intestine which extends from the cecum to the rectum.

Congenital: Existing at or dating from birth.

Contrecoup: Injury resulting from a blow on a remote part.

Contusion: Bruise as a result of rupture of the blood vessels.

Convulsion: A violent, involuntary contraction or series of contractions of the voluntary muscles.

Coronary: A term applied to vessels, nerves, ligaments.

Corpse: The dead body of a human being.

Corpus delicti: The body of a crime. The substantial fact that a crime has been committed.

Corroborate: To add credibility by additional and confirming evidence or facts.

Cranium: The skull or brain pan.

Crime: An offense against the state, punishable by imprisonment or fine or both.

Culpable: Blamable.

Cyanosis: Blueness of the skin, often due to cardiac malformation causing insufficient oxygenation of the blood (increase in carboxyhemoglobin).

Dead: Without life.

Deadly weapon: Any instrument or weapon which from the manner used is calculated or likely to produce death or great bodily harm.

Decomposition: The separation of compound bodies into their constituent principles—post-mortem degeneration of the body.

Degeneration: Deterioration.

Delirium: A mental disorder marked by illusions, hallucinations, physical restlessness and incoherence.

Dentine: The chief substance or tissue of the teeth which surrounds the tooth pulp; resembles bone.

Depraved: Perverted.

Deteriorate: To become worse—impairment.

Diabetes: A disease characterized by insufficient insulin action usually accompanied by the passage of sugar in the urine, or a deficiency condition marked by habitual discharge of an excessive quantity of urine.

Diagnosis: The art of distinguishing one disease from another.

Diaphragm: The musculomembranous partition that separates the abdomen from the thorax.

Disarticulation: Amputation or separation at a joint.

Disease: Any departure from a state of health; illness or sickness.

Disinterment: Digging up body after burial.

Distal: Remote, farthest from the center.

Dorsal: Pertaining to the back .

Dotage: Feebleness of mind in old age.

Duodenum: The first portion of the small intestine.

Dysentery: A term given to a number of disorders marked by inflammation of the intestines, and attended by pain in the abdomen and frequent stools containing blood and mucus.

Ecto: A prefix denoting situated on, without, or on the outside.

Eczema: An inflammatory skin disease.

Edema: The presence of abnormally large amounts of fluid in the intercellular tissue spaces of the body.

Ejaculation: A sudden act of expulsion, as of semen.

Embalming: The treatment of the dead body to prevent putrefaction.

Embolism: A blocking of an artery or vein by a clot or obstruction (usually carried by blood circulation).

Embryo: The fetus in its earlier stages of development.

Epidermis: The outermost layer of the skin.

Epilepsy: A chronic functional disease characterized by brief convulsive seizures in which there is loss of consciousness, with a succession of tonic or clonic convulsions.

Evidence: Any species of proof legally presented at a trial.

Exit wound: The wound made by a weapon where it emerges from and after passing completely through the body, or any part of it.

Excrement: Matter cast out as waste from the body.

Exhibitionism: A perversion of the sexual feeling that leads an individual to expose his genital organs in public.

Expert: Witnesses in a cause who are permitted to give their opinions on some professional or technical matter because of their special training or familiarity with it.

Extenuate: To lessen.

Extra: A prefix meaning outside of, beyond, or in addition.

Exhume: The disinterring or removal of a body from the grave.

Eyewitness: A person who saw the act or transaction to which he testifies.

Fatal injury: An injury resulting in death.

Felonious homicide: The killing of a human being without justification or excuse.

Felony: A crime carrying a punishment of imprisonment in the penitentiary.

Femur: The thigh bone.

Fetishism: Association of lust with items of certain portions of the female body or with certain articles of female attire.

Fetus: The unborn offspring of a human or an animal.

Firearm: A weapon which employs gunpowder to fire a projectile.

Fistula: An ulcer, often leading to an internal hollow organ.

Force: Unlawful violence.

Fratricide: The act of killing one's brother or sister.

Gangrene: Death of tissue, characterized by anoxia and marked inflammation.

Hemorrhage: Bleeding.

Histotoxic: Poisonous to tissue or tissues.

Homicidomania: Impulsive desire to commit murder.

Homosexual: Sex acts or feelings directed toward a person of the same sex.

Hydrophobia: The usual common name for rabies in man.

Hypertension: High blood pressure.

Identity: The fact that a person or thing is the same as it is represented to be.

Incision: A wound inflicted by an instrument with a sharp cutting edge.

Incompetency: Inadequacy or insufficiency.

Incriminate: To charge with a crime.

Infanticide: The act of killing an infant soon after birth.

Infarct: An area of necrosis (death of a cell or group of cells) in a tissue produced by sudden arrest of circulation in a vessel.

> **Myocardia infarction:** An area of death in heart tissue, usually resulting from coronary thrombosis.

> **Pulmonary infarction:** An area of necrosis in lung tissue produced by sudden arrest of circulation in a vessel.

Inhalation: The drawing of air or other vapor into the lungs.

Insane: Unsound in mind.

Intent: Purpose.

Interstitial: Pertaining to or situated in the interstices or interspaces of a tissue.

Intestine: The membranous tube that extends from the stomach to the anus.

Intra: Prefix meaning within.

Kill: To deprive of life.

Laceration: A split or tear of the skin, produced usually by blunt force.

Latent: Concealed; hidden.

Lateral: Pertaining to a side.

Legally: According to law.

Ligament: Any fibrous, tough band which connects bones or supports viscera.

Ligature: Anything that binds or ties.

Liver: A large gland situated in the upper part of the abdomen on the right side, usually of a dark red color.

Lividity: Post-mortem discoloration by the gravitation of blood.

Lumbar: Pertaining to or near the lower region of the back.

Maim: To disable by a wound.

Malice: The doing of a wrongful act intentionally without just cause or excuse.

Malice aforethought: The preconceived intent to commit a murder or any other felony.

Manslaughter: The unlawful killing of another without malice and without premeditation and without deliberation.

> **Involuntary:** Killing of another as a result of carelessness or recklessness, such as doing an act which is unlawful but not felonious, or by doing a lawful act without proper caution or skill.

> **Voluntary:** Killing of another without a design to effect death or without malice, express or implied, such as in "heat of blood" or "by provocation."

Masochism: Sexual perversion in which the pervert takes delight in being subjected to degrading, humiliating or cruel treatment such as flogging or choking.

Masturbation: Sexual self-abuse and/or gratification.

Mayhem: The act of unlawfully and violently depriving another of the use of members or parts of his body.

Medial: Pertaining to the middle.

Membrane: A thin layer of tissue which covers a surface or divides a space or organ.

Meningitis: Inflammation of the meninges (thin membranous coverings of brain).

Mental capacity: The measure of intelligence or understanding as will enable a person to understand the nature of his acts.

Miscarriage: The premature emptying of a uterus prior to 28 weeks of gestation.

Misdemeanor: Criminal offense which does not amount to a felony, punishable by a term in the city or county jail up to one year, or a fine, or both.

Monomania: Insanity on a single subject or class of subjects.

Mortuary: A place where dead bodies are kept for a time before burial.

Motive: The cause or reason why a thing is done.

Mummification: The complete drying up of the body as the result of burial in a dry place, or by exposure to dry atmosphere.

Murder: The crime committed by a person of sound mind and discretion, old enough to formulate and execute a criminal design, without any justification or excuse, with malice aforethought, provided that death results from the injury inflicted within one year and a day after its infliction.

First Degree Murder:

   A. Murder by means of poison, or by lying in wait or any other kind of willful or premeditated killing.

   B. Murder committed in the perpetration of or attempted perpetration of any felony, such as rape, burglary, arson, mayhem or robbery.

Second Degree Murder: The intentional killing of another willfully and maliciously.

   Note: Deliberation is the determining factor between 1st and 2nd Degree Murder. It is essential in Murder in the 1st Degree. Deliberation may be defined as "done in a cool state of blood" and not in sudden passion or caused by just provocation.

Myocardium: The heart muscle.

Narcomania: An insane desire for narcotics or alcohol.

Natal: Pertains to birth.

Nausea: Tendency to vomit; sickness at the stomach.

Necessity, Homicide by: Justifiable homicide; arises without any intention or desire and without any negligence or inadvertence on the part of the person doing the killing, and therefore without blame.

Necrophilism: Morbid attraction to corpses; sexual intercourse with a dead body.

Negligence: The omission to do something which a reasonable man guided by those ordinary considerations which ordinarily regulate human affairs would do, or the doing of something which a reasonable and prudent man would not do.

Criminal Negligence: Negligence of such a character, or occurring under such circumstances as to be punishable as a crime.

Gross Negligence: Willful and wanton negligence; a higher degree of negligence than ordinary negligence.

Wanton Negligence: Reckless indifference to the consequences of an act or omission.

Willful Negligence: Same as wanton; used sometimes to describe a degree of negligence higher than gross.

Next of kin: Persons most nearly related to the deceased by blood.

Non compos mentis: Not sound of mind; insane.

Nymphomania: Exaggerated sexual desire in a female.

Offense: A breach of the criminal law.

Organ: A part of the body having a specific function.

Ossification: Formation of bone or a bony substance.

Osteitis: Inflammation of a bone.

Osteomyelitis: Inflammation of bone caused by pyogenic organism.

Ovary: The female sexual organ (gonads) in which the ova (eggs) are formed.

Overt: Open.

Pancreas: A large elongated gland behind the stomach.

Papillary: Pertaining to or resembling a nipple, ridges or grooves.

Paralysis: The loss of the power of voluntary motion.

Paranoia: A mental disorder characterized by the development of ambitions or suspicions into delusions of persecution.

Parenticide: The act of killing one's own parents.

Passion: As used in the criminal law, the term means intense and vehement emotional excitement prompting aggressive and violent action.

Patent: Open.

Pathology: The part of medicine which explains the nature, cause and symptoms of diseases.

Patricide: The act of murdering one's own father.

Pederasty: Sexual intercourse with boys by the anus.

Penetration: The insertion of the male part into the female parts to however slight an extent.

Penis: The male organ of copulation.

Percussion: The act of striking a part with short, sharp blows.

Permeation: The spreading through a tissue or organ of a disease process.

Petechial hemorrhages: Hemorrhages that occur in minute (pinlike) points beneath the skin.

Phalanx: Any bone of a finger or toe.

Phonomania: Insanity marked by a tendency to commit murder.

Physical: Relating to or pertaining to the body.

Pneumatic: Pertaining to air or respiration.

Poisons:
- (1) Gases
- (2) Anesthetics
- (3) Corrosives
    - (a) Strong mineral acids
    - (b) Strong alkalies
- (4) Metallic poisons
- (5) Organic poisons
    - (a) Alkaloids
    - (b) Non-alkaloids
- (6) Food poisons.

Polygraph: Instrument for measuring the pulse.

Post-mortem: After death.

Pregnancy: The condition of having a developing embryo or fetus in the body.

Probable cause: An apparent state of facts, upon reasonable inquiry, found to exist, which would induce a reasonable and prudent man to believe that the person charged has committed the crime.

Prohibit: To prevent or forbid by law.

Proximal: Nearest to the center.

Proximate cause: That which, in a natural and continuous sequence, unbroken by any intervening cause, produces the injury, and without which the result would not have occurred.

Psychoanalysis: The method of eliciting from patients past emotional experiences in order to discover the mechanism by which a pathologic mental state has been produced.

Psychosomatic: Pertaining to the mind-body relationship.

Pubic: Pertaining to the pubes (anterior pelvic bones).

Pulmonary: Pertaining to the lungs.

Pulmonary embolism: The closure of the pulmonary artery or one of its branches by an embolus.

Putrefaction: Decomposition of soft tissues by bacteria and enzymes.

Rancid: Having a musty, rank taste or smell.

Rape: Sexual intercourse with any female under the age of 16 years, or with a female over 16 years forcibly and against her will.

Reasonable and probable cause: Such grounds as would justify a reasonable and prudent man to believe that a certain set of facts are as they appear to be.

Recognizance: Bond to guarantee appearance.

Relevancy: Related to the crime.

Remote cause: A cause which does not cause the effect intended due to the intervening of a proximate cause.

Respiration: The act or function of breathing.

Retardation: Delay or hindrance.

Rigor mortis: A rigidity or stiffening of the muscular tissue and joints of the body after death.

Sacro: Combining form denoting relationship to the sacrum.

Sadism: Sexual perversion in which satisfaction is derived from the infliction of cruelty upon another.

Sane: Normal and healthy mental condition.

Sanguine: Abounding in blood.

Schizophrenia: A mental disorder.

Sclerosis: Induration or hardening.

Self-defense: The protection of one's person or property against some injury by another.

Semen: The thick, whitish secretion of the reproductive organs in the male.

Senile: Pertaining to old age.

Sororicide: Act of murdering one's sister.

Spasm: Sudden, violent, involuntary contraction of a muscle or group of muscles.

Sputum: Matter ejected from the mouth; saliva and mucus.

Stagnant: Failure of circulation (for example, shock, cardiac failure).

Stillbirth: 28 weeks of gestation, or over, born dead.

Strangulation: Any abnormal constriction of the throat, such as causes a suspension of breathing.

Strepho: Combining form meaning twisted.

Stroke: A sudden or severe attack, with rupture of the blood vessel.

Suffocation: The stoppage of respiration.

Suicide: Self destruction; the deliberate taking of one's own life.

Tarsus: The instep proper of the foot with its seven bones.

Tetanus: An acute infectious disease caused by bacteria which release a powerful toxin.

Thermo: Combining form denoting relationship to heat.

Thrombo: Combining form denoting relationship to a clot.

Tibia: The inner and larger bone of the leg below the knee.

Tissue: An aggregation of cells united in the performance of a particular function.

Torso: The trunk of the body without the head or extremities.

Toxic: Poisonous.

Toxicologist: An expert in the knowledge and detection of poisons.

Trachea: The windpipe.

Tranquilizer: Medication having quieting or calming effect.

Trauma: A wound or injury.

Tremor: An involuntary trembling or quivering.

Ultimate: Facts in issue.

Umbilical: Pertaining to the umbilicus (navel).

Unlawful: That which is contrary or unauthorized by law.

Urine: The fluid secreted by the kidneys, stored in the bladder and discharged by the urethra.

Uterus: The womb.

Vaginal: Pertaining to the vagina (female sexual canal).

Vascular: Pertaining to or full of vessels.

Vein: A vein which conveys the blood to or toward the heart.

Ventricle: One of the two lower cavities of the heart.

Voltage: Electric force.

Wanton: Reckless disregard for the safety of others.

Willful murder: The unlawful and intentional killing of another without just cause or excuse.

Wound: An injury to the person caused by physical means with disruption of the normal continuity of body structures (breaking of the skin).

—43—

INTERNATIONAL CLASSIFICATION
OF CAUSES OF DEATH

I. Violent or accidental deaths
    A.   Suicide by solid or liquid poisons, or by poison-
        ous gases
        1. Arsenic and compounds
        2. Barbituric acid and derivatives
        3. Cresol compounds
        4. Mercury and compounds
        5. Nux vomica and strychnine
        6. Carbolic acid and phenol
        7. Other solid or liquid poisons
        8. Illuminating gas
        9. Motor vehicle exhaust gas
      10. Other carbon monoxide gas
      11. Other poisonous gases
    B.   Suicide by other means
        1. Hanging or strangulation
        2. Drowning
        3. Firearms and explosives
        4. Cutting or piercing instruments
        5. Jumping from high places
        6. Crushing
        7. Other unspecified means
    C.   Infanticide
        Killing of an infant

D. Homicide by
    1. Firearms
    2. Cutting or piercing instruments
    3. By other means
E. Railway accidents (except collisions with motor vehicles)
F. Motor vehicle accidents
    1. Collisions between automobiles and trains
    2. Collisions between automobiles and street-cars
    3. Automobile accidents (except collisions with trains or street-cars)
    4. Motorcycle accidents (except collisions with automobiles)
G. Street-car and other road-transport accidents
    1. Street-car accidents (except collisions with trains or motor vehicles)
    2. Other and unspecified road transport accidents
H. Water-transport accidents
I. Air-transport accidents
J. Accidents in mines and quarries
K. Agricultural and forestry accidents
    1. Involving agricultural machinery and vehicles
    2. Injury by animals in agriculture
    3. Other agricultural accidents
    4. Involving forestry machinery and vehicles
    5. Other forestry accidents
L. Other accidents involving machinery
M. Food poisoning
N. Accidental absorption of poisonous gas
    1. Illuminating gas
    2. Motor vehicle exhaust gas

        3. Other carbon monoxide gas
        4. Other poisonous gases

O.   Acute accidental poisoning by solids or liquids
        1. Arsenic and compounds
        2. Barbituric acid and derivatives
        3. Cresol compounds
        4. Mercury and compounds
        5. Nux vomica and strychnine
        6. Carbolic acid and phenol
        7. Lye and potash
        8. Tobacco and derivatives
        9. Narcotics
      10. Methanol and other alcohols
      11. Other and unspecified substances

Q.   Conflagration

P.   Accidental burns (except due to conflagration)

R.   Accidental mechanical suffocation

S.   Accidental drowning

T.   Accidental injury by firearms

U.   Accidental injury by cutting or piercing instruments

V.   Accidental injury by fall or crushing
        1. Fall
        2. Crushing

W.   Cataclysm (all deaths attributed to a cataclysm regardless of their nature)

X.   Injury by animals (not specified as venomous or occupying in the course of agricultural and forestry operations

Y.   Hunger or thirst

Z.   Excessive cold

AA. Excessive heat

BB. Lightning

CC. Accidents due to electric currents (except lightning)

DD. Poisoning by venomous animals (not specified as occurring in the course of agricultural and forestry operations)

EE. Other accidents
1. Sequelae of preventive immunization, inoculation or vaccination
2. Other accidents due to medical or surgical intervention
3. Lack of care of the new-born
4. Obstruction, suffocation or puncture by ingested objects
5. Other and unspecified accidents

FF. Deaths of military personnel during operations of war

GG. Deaths of civilians due to operations of war

HH. Legal executions

II. Ill-defined and unknown causes
A. Sudden death
B. Ill-defined or unknown causes
1. Ill-defined
2. Found dead (cause unknown)
3. Unknown or unspecified (natural) cause
Note: All of the above should be considered deaths requiring investigation and reporting to the Coroner's Office

—44—

GUIDE TO APPENDIX

Illustrations of parts of body   Forms #1 — #11
- # 1   Human skeleton
- # 2   Human Body
- # 3   Head and facial bones
- # 4   Digestive system (frontal view)
- # 5   Digestive system (back view)
- # 6   Breathing system
- # 7   Hand
- # 8   Foot
- # 9   Heart
- #10   Brain
- #11   Eye

Identification of guns   Forms #12 — #15
- #12   Types of small arms and weapons
- #13   Most commonly used small arms
- #14   Shotgun
- #15   Rifle

Firearm distance chart	Form #16
Body Burn Percentage Chart	Form #17
Vehicle Stopping Distance Chart	Forms #18, #18a
Photograph Data	Form #19
Sketch and Diagraming Symbols	Form #20
Teeth (Dental) Charts	Forms #21 & #22
Investigation Reports	Forms #23 — #38

- #23   Poisons
- #24   Gunshot
- #25   Hanging
- #26   Auto
- #27   Apparent Natural

#28 Under the Influence of Liquor
#29 Clothing & Personal Effects
#30 Clothing Record
#31 Money and Valuables Record
#32 Report of Missing Person
#33 General Physical Appearance Report
#34 Interim Report to Law Enforcement Agency
#35 Toxicological Examination Report
#36 X-ray Report
#37 Medico-Legal Report
#38 Report to Accompany Body to Morgue

Evidence Collection Chart   Form #39
Receipts for Possessions and Evidence   Form #40
Record of phone calls and inquiries   Form #41
Standard Death Certificate   Form #42
Fetal Death Certificate   Form #43
Autopsy Consent Form   Form #44
Poison Chart   Form #45
Fetus (Determination of Age)   Form #46
Stain Field Test   Forms #47 — #49

#47 Benzidine Test for Blood
#48 Firearms Residue Identification
#49 Paraffin Residue Identification

FORMS

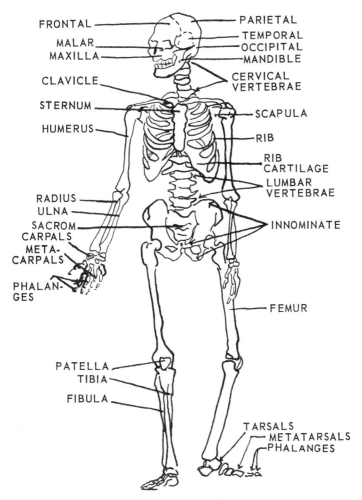

Form 1. Human skeleton.

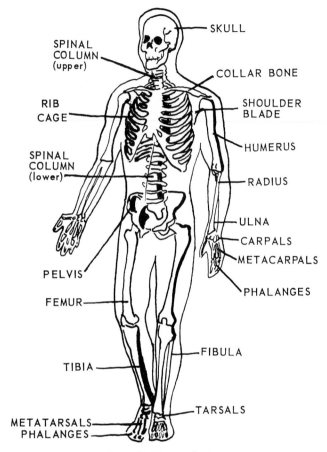

Form 2. Human body.

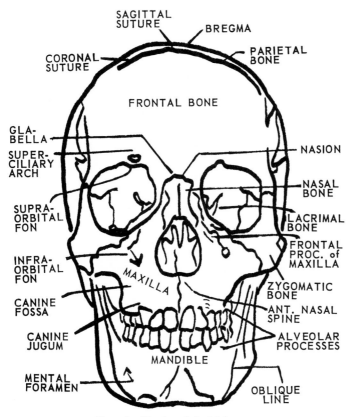

Form 3. Head and facial bones.

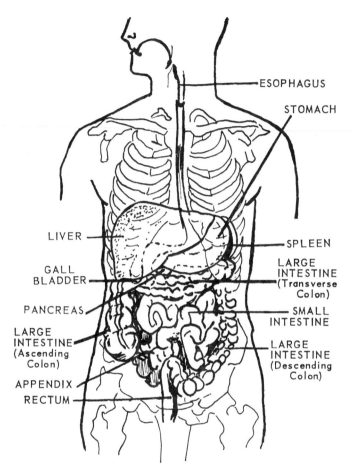

Form 4. Digestive system (frontal view).

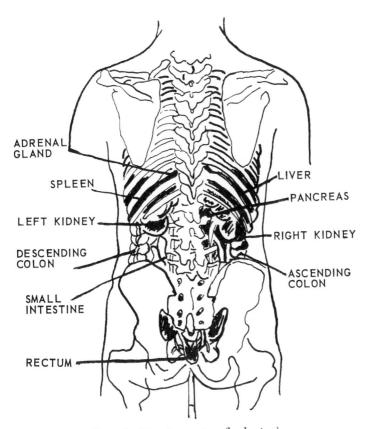

Form 5. Digestive system (back view).

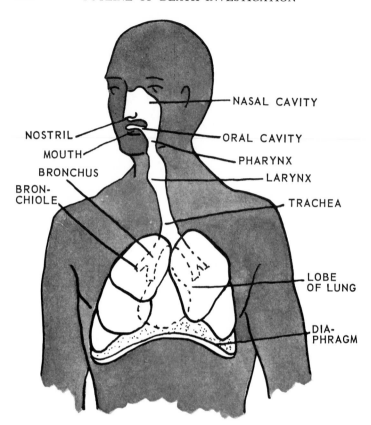

Form 6. Breathing system.

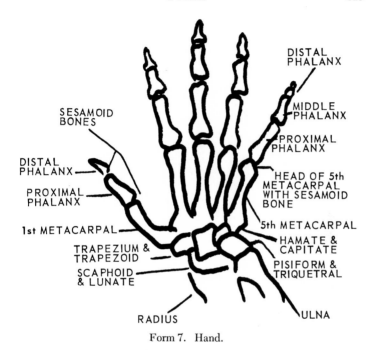

Form 7. Hand.

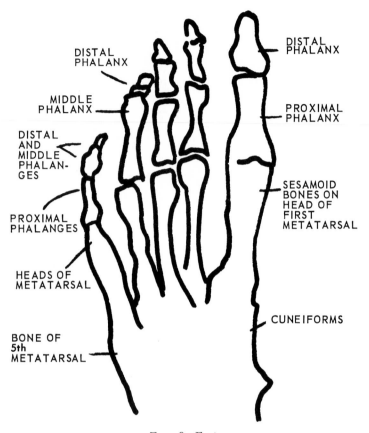

Form 8.   Foot.

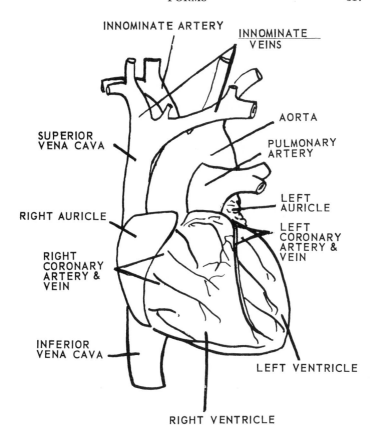

INNOMINATE ARTERY

INNOMINATE
VEINS

AORTA

SUPERIOR
VENA CAVA

PULMONARY
ARTERY

LEFT
AURICLE

RIGHT AURICLE

LEFT
CORONARY
ARTERY &
VEIN

RIGHT
CORONARY
ARTERY &
VEIN

INFERIOR
VENA CAVA

LEFT VENTRICLE

RIGHT VENTRICLE

HEART AND MAJOR BLOOD VESSELS

Form 9.   Heart.

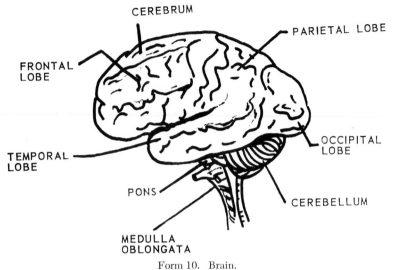

CEREBRUM

PARIETAL LOBE

FRONTAL
LOBE

OCCIPITAL
LOBE

TEMPORAL
LOBE

PONS

CEREBELLUM

MEDULLA
OBLONGATA

Form 10. Brain.

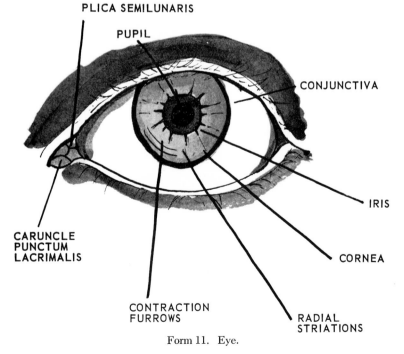

PLICA SEMILUNARIS

PUPIL

CONJUNCTIVA

CARUNCLE
PUNCTUM
LACRIMALIS

IRIS

CORNEA

CONTRACTION
FURROWS

RADIAL
STRIATIONS

Form 11. Eye.

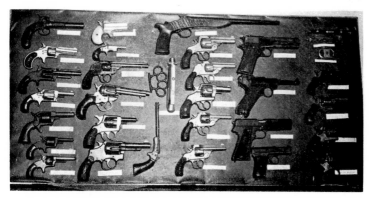

Form 12. Types of small arms and weapons.

Types of Guns and Weapons

1st Row, top to bottom:

Cap and Ball—35 cal.
Derringer—32 cal. single action
Smith & Wesson rim fire, 32 cal.
Defender—rim fire—32 cal.
Allen & Wheelcock—32 cal.—rim fire
Prairie—22 cal.—rim fire
Hopkins & Allen—22 cal. rim fire

2nd Row, top to bottom:

Derringer—41 cal., over & under
Derringer—22 cal.
Forehand, Hammerless, 32 cal.,
    center fire
Colt 38—Western
H & R—22 cal.
Smith & Wesson—38 cal. Police Spec.

3rd Row, top to bottom:

410 Shotgun pistol
Brass knuckles
Spring knife
Derringer 22 target pistol

4th Row, top to bottom:

Harrington & Richards 38 cal.
    short—1887
Forehand Arms, 32 cal.—1887
American Double Action 45 cal., center
    fire, 1891
Double action 32 cal., rim fire, 1899
Hopkins & Allen 32 cal., center fire 1861

5th Row, top to bottom:

Colt automatic, 45 cal. W. W. #1
9 MM Luger "German," Grasshopper
    Action—1914
Radom—"German," 38 cal.—1941
Mauser "German," 25 cal. 1914

6th Row, top to bottom:

Gas pocket gun
Thumb cuffs
"English" 32 cal.—1885
"English" Rev. 32 cal., pin-fire
38 cal. center fire—1873
Bull dog, 38 cal.

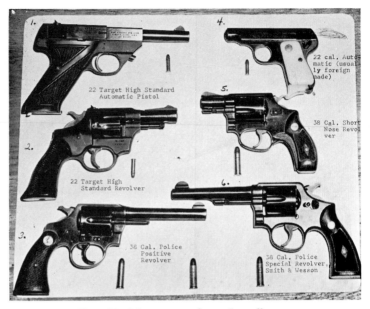

Form 13. Most commonly used small arms.

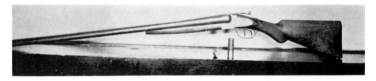

Form 14. Shotgun.

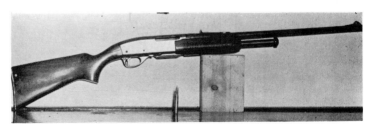

Form 15. Rifle.

CONTUSION RING   POWDER

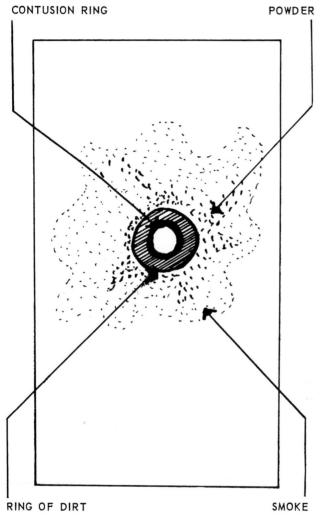

RING OF DIRT   SMOKE

Form 16.   Firearm distance chart.

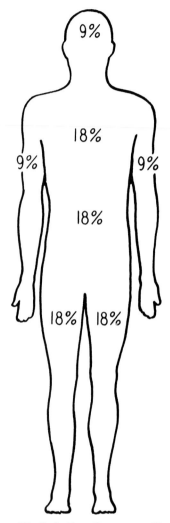

Form 17. Body Burn Percentage Chart.

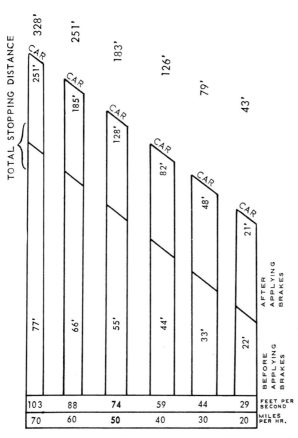

Form 18. Vehicle Stopping Distance Chart.

SPEED, TIME AND DISTANCE TABLES

Distance = Speed X Time.

Time = $\dfrac{\text{Distances}}{\text{Speed}}$

Speed = $\dfrac{\text{Distances}}{\text{Time}}$

5280 feet equals one mile. A vehicle traveling at the rate of one mile per hour will cover a distance of 1.4666 feet per second. A vehicle traveling at the rate of twelve miles per hour will cover a distance twelve times 1.4666 or 17.590 feet in one second.

A person walking slowly will cover a distance of two miles per hour or 2.933 feet per second. A person walking at a moderate gait will cover a distance of about three miles per hour or about 4.39 feet in one second. A person walking rapidly will cover a distance of four miles per hour or 5.866 feet per second.

The following table shows the distances in feet covered in one second at various rates of speed.

SPEED AND DISTANCE TABLE

Rate of Speed Miles Per Hour	Feet Covered in One Second DISTANCE	Rate of Speed Miles Per Hour	Feet Covered in One Second DISTANCE
1	1.4666	26	38.1316
2	2.9332	27	39.5982
3	4.3998	28	41.0648
4	5.8664	29	42.5314
5	7.333	30	43.998
6	8.7996	31	45.4646
7	10.2662	32	46.9312
8	11.7328	33	48.3978
9	13.1994	34	49.8644
10	14.666	35	51.331
11	16.1326	36	52.7976
12	17.5992	37	54.2642
13	19.0658	38	55.7308
14	20.5324	39	57.1974
15	21.999	40	58.664
16	23.4656	41	60.1306
17	24.9322	42	61.5968
18	26.3988	43	63.0638
19	27.8654	44	64.5304
20	29.332	45	65.997
21	30.7986	46	67.4636
22	32.2652	47	68.9302
23	33.7318	48	70.3968
24	35.1984	49	71.8634
25	36.665	50	73.33

Form 18a. Vehicle Stopping Distance Chart.

This Photograph the Property
Coroner's Office
St. Louis County, Missouri

Date_____ Time_____

Subject _____

Case No._____

Location _____

Taken By_____

Shutter_____ Lens_____

Process Date _____

Processed By_____

Distance From Subject_____

Form 19. Photograph Data.

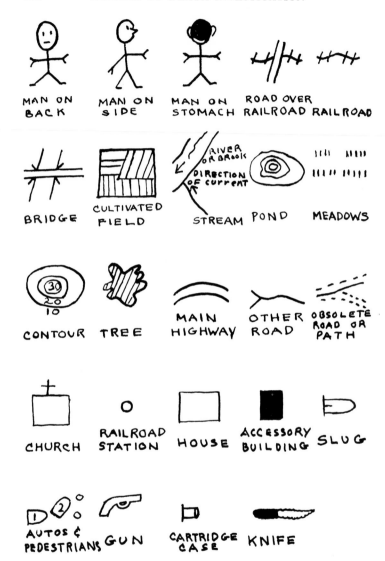

Form 20. Sketch and Diagraming Symbols.

© 1960 PROFESSIONAL BUDGET PLAN   MADISON, WIS.

LAST NAME	FIRST NAME	RECOMMENDED BY	NAME OF PHYSICIAN
ADDRESS		ADDRESS	ADDRESS OR TELEPHONE
CITY	STATE	REFERRED TO OR BY DR.	DATE OF EXAMINATION

| 1 | 2 | 3 | 4 | 5 | 6 | 7 | 8 | | 9 | 10 | 11 | 12 | 13 | 14 | 15 | 16 |
| 8 | 7 | 6 | 5 | 4 | 3 | 2 | 1 | 1 | 2 | 3 | 4 | 5 | 6 | 7 | 8 |

X-rays _____
Date _____
Study Model _____
Photograph _____
Transillumination
Area _____

MOULD

calculus deposits Slight? _____ Moderate? _____ Excessive? _____

TOOTH	Upper	Lower
Central		
Lateral		
Cuspid		
Posteriors		

SHADE

TOOTH	Upper	Lower
Central		
Lateral		
Cuspid		
Posteriors		

| 8 | 7 | 6 | 5 | 4 | 3 | 2 | 1 | 1 | 2 | 3 | 4 | | 5 | 6 | 7 | 8 |
| 32 | 31 | 30 | 29 | 28 | 27 | 26 | 25 | 24 | 23 | 22 | 21 | 20 | 19 | 18 | 17 |

HEALTH HISTORY

What is the general condition of teeth? _____

What is the general condition of soft tissue? _____ Color? _____

Inflammation present? _____ Moderate? _____ Severe? _____ Condition of saliva? ____

Is there any recession? _____ Is there any pain in the region of the ear? _____

Do you have difficulty hearing? _____ Abnormalities _____

How is the occlusion? _____ Attitude _____

How long since you have been to a dentist? _____ What was done then? _____

Did you have x-rays? _____ Did you make regular visits to the dentist before then? _____

Have you lost many teeth? _____ Why? _____

Were there any complications with the extractions? _____

Have they ever been replaced by: A fixed bridge? _____ A removable partial? _____ A denture? _____

How often do you brush your teeth? _____ When? _____

Do the gums bleed? _____ When? _____

Does food collect between your teeth? _____ Is your breath offensive? _____

Do you eat sweets? _____ Raw vegetables? _____ Do you eat between meals? _____

Do you have excessive bleeding from a cut? _____ Date of birth? _____

Are your teeth sensitive to heat? _____ To cold? _____ To sweets? _____

When was your last complete physical examination? _____ Weight? _____

Are you under the care of a physician now? _____ For what reason? _____

Are you receiving any medication? _____ What? _____

Have you ever had radiation treatment? _____ Anemia? _____ Diabetes? _____

Do you have any allergies? _____ Penicillin? _____ Novocain? _____ Food? _____

Arthritis? _____ Rheumatic fever? _____ Abnormal blood pressure? _____ Heart condition? _____

Have you ever had hepatitis? _____ T.B.? _____ Comments: _____

_____

_____

_____ Form No. 98D

Form 21. Teeth (Dental) Chart.

OUTLINE OF DEATH INVESTIGATION

© 1956 PROFESSIONAL BUDGET PLAN   MADISON, WIS.

LAST NAME   FIRST NAME   RECOMMENDED BY   NAME OF PHYSICIAN

ADDRESS   ADDRESS   ADDRESS OR TELEPHONE

CITY   STATE   REFERRED TO OR BY DR   NO. OF PATIENT

1	2	3	4	5	6	7	8	9	10	11	12	13	14	15	16
8	7	6	5	4	3	2	1	1	2	3	4	5	6	7	8

MOULD

TOOTH	Upper	Lower
Central		
Lateral		
Cuspid		
Posteriors		

SHADE

TOOTH	Upper	Lower
Central		
Lateral		
Cuspid		
Posteriors		

X-Rays_____
Date_____
Study Model_____
Date_____
Photograph_____
Date_____
Transillumination
Area_____

8	7	6	5	4	3	2	1	1	2	3	4	5	6	7	8
32	31	30	29	28	27	26	25	24	23	22	21	20	19	18	17

V	IV	III	II	I	I	II	III	IV	V

E	D	C	B	A	A	B	C	D	E

School_____ Grade_____
Tonsils_____ Adenoids_____
Diseases — Measles_____ Chickenpox_____
Scarlet fever_____ Whooping cough_____
Mumps_____ Other_____
Habits — Thumb or finger sucking_____ Posture_____
Mouth breathing_____ Tongue_____
Reaction to dentistry_____

HEALTH HISTORY

What is the general condition of teeth?_____
What is the general condition of soft tissue?_____ Color?_____
Inflammation present?_____ Moderate?_____ Severe?_____ Condition of saliva?_____
Is there any recession?_____ Is there any pain in the region of the ear?_____
Calculus deposits?_____ Slight?_____ Moderate?_____ Excessive?_____
How is the occlusion?_____ Attitude_____
How long since you have been to a dentist?_____ What was done then?_____
Did you have x-rays?_____ Did you make regular visits to the dentist before then?_____
Have you lost many teeth?_____ Why?_____
Were there any complications with the extractions?_____
Have they ever been replaced by A fixed bridge?_____ A removable partial?_____ A denture?_____
If patient says no, "Have you ever been told what might happen if lost teeth are not replaced?"_____
How often do you brush your teeth?_____ When?_____
Do the gums bleed when you brush your teeth?_____ Do they bleed at other times?_____
Does food collect between your teeth?_____ Do you have bad breath?_____
Do you eat between meals?_____ Sweets?_____ Raw vegetables?_____
Do you have excessive bleeding from a cut?_____ Date of birth?_____
Are your teeth sensitive to heat?_____ To cold?_____ To sweets?_____
How long since you have had a complete physical examination?_____
Are you under the care of a physician now?_____ For what reason?_____
Are you receiving any medication?_____ What?_____
Have you ever had x-ray therapy?_____ Anemia?_____ Diabetes?_____
Do you have any allergies?_____ Penicillin?_____ Novocain?_____
Arthritis?_____ Rheumatic fever?_____ Blood pressure?_____ Heart trouble?_____

_____
_____ Form No. 76

Form 22. Teeth (Dental) Chart.

INVESTIGATION REPORT

Name_____(m) (f) (w) (c) Age_____

Address_____ City_____

Marital Status_____ Occupation_____

Nearest Relative_____ Telephone No._____

Date_____ Time _____ How Rec'd._____

How and by whom reported_____

Scene _____ _____

How clothed _____

When found_____ By whom found_____

Body location (sketch attached)_____

IF MEDICATION, LIST THE FOLLOWING	**IF CARBON MONOXIDE, LIST PROBABLE SOURCE**
Type of Medication	
Name of prescribing physician	
Name of pharmacist	
Date prescribed	
Quantity prescribed	
Quantity missing	
To whom prescribed	
Location of containers	

Description of premises_____

Condition of premises_____

Suicide note_____ (Contents of note—see attached sheet)

Handwriting identified by_____

Apparent reason _____

When seen last_____ By whom_____

Where_____Subject matter of last conversation

Previous threats_____ To whom made_____

Previous attempts_____ How_____ When_____

Other persons at premises at time of occurrence_____

Form 23. Poisons. Actual size 8½ x 13.

INVESTIGATION REPORT – GUNSHOT

Name_____(m) (f) (w) (c) Age_____
Address_____ City_____
Marital Status_____ Occupation_____
Nearest Relative_____ Telephone No._____
Date_____ Time _____ How Rec'd._____
How and by whom reported_____
Scene _____
How clothed _____
When found_____ By whom found_____
Body and gun location (Sketch attached)_____

SMALL ARM:	RIFLE:	SHOTGUN:
Type	Type	Type
Make	Make	Make
Caliber	Single shot	Gauge
Discharged slugs in gun	Automatic	Length of barrel
Not discharged in gun	Length of barrel	"Shot"
Location of spent cartridge	Caliber	Discharged
	Discharged	Not discharged
	Not discharged	Automatic or single shot

Blood stains (location)_____
_____ (Wet)_____ (Dried)_____ (Semi-dried)_____
Subject: Ownership
(R.H._____) (L.H._____) of gun_____
Usual location where gun is kept_____
Gun identified by whom_____
Description of premises _____
Condition of premises_____
Suicide note_____ (Contents of note—see attached sheet)
Handwriting identified by_____
Apparent reason _____
                                     By
When seen last_____ whom_____
Where_____Subject matter of last conversation
_____
                            To whom
Previous Threats_____ made_____
Previous attempts_____ How_____ When_____
Other persons at premises at apparent time of shooting_____

Form 24. Gunshot. Actual size 8½ x 13.

INVESTIGATION REPORT — HANGING

Name_____(m) (f) (w) (c) Age_____

Address _____ City_____

Marital Status_____ Occupation_____

Nearest Relative_____ Telephone No._____

Date_____ Time_____ How Rec'd._____

How and by whom reported_____

Scene _____

How clothed _____

When found _____

By whom found_____

Body location (sketch attached)_____

Position of body _____

    Height from which suspended_____

    Suspended from where_____

                                    Distance

Platform_____ Type_____ Height_____from body_____

                               Obtained

Type of ligature used_____ from_____

Length of ligature_____ How tied_____

Location of knot_____

                           Deceased:

Body cut down by whom_____(R.H.) (L.H.)

Description of premises _____

    Condition of premises_____

Suicide note_____(Contents of note—See attached sheet).

Handwriting identified by_____

Apparent reason _____

When seen last _____

    By whom_____ Where_____

    Subject matter of last conversation_____

Previous threats_____ To whom made_____

Previous attempts_____ How_____ When_____

Other persons at premises at apparent time of hanging_____

REMARKS: _____

Form 25. Hanging. Actual size 8½ x 13.

ACCIDENT REPORT

DEPARTMENT OF POLICE
ST. LOUIS COUNTY, MISSOURI

CLAYTON 5, MISSOURI

Complaint No. _____

District _____

Log Point _____

Highway _____

Date _____

LOCATION   In City of _____ at _____ Time _____ AM PM _____
(INTERSECTING STREET)

of

ACCIDENT   In _____ County _____ Miles of _____
Feet (DIRECTION) (INTERSECTING STATE HIGHWAY, COUNTY LINE OR CITY LIMIT)

CAR NUMBER 1: _____ _____ _____ Registration _____ _____ _____
(YEAR) (MAKE) (TYPE, AS SEDAN, CAB, TRUCK, BUS, ETC.) (YEAR) (STATE) (NUMBER)

Driven by _____ Lic.No. _____
(NAME) (STREET ADDRESS) (CITY & STATE) CHAUFFER OPERATOR

Owned by _____
(NAME) (STREET ADDRESS) (CITY & STATE)

Driver's Age _____ Sex _____ Color _____ Driving Exp. ____ Years. Dir.of Travel _____ Speed _____
(OFFICER'S EST)

Driver's Occupation _____ Has driver had High School driver training _____
Place of Employment _____ Address _____
Speed Limit _____ Damage to Car _____ Estimated Amount $ _____
Statement of Driver _____
_____
_____

CAR NUMBER 2: _____ _____ _____ Registration _____ _____ _____
(YEAR) (MAKE) (TYPE, AS SEDAN, CAB, TRUCK, BUS, ETC.) (YEAR) (STATE) (NUMBER)

Driven by _____ Lic.No. _____
(NAME) (STREET ADDRESS) (CITY & STATE) CHAUFFER OPERATOR

Owned by _____
(NAME) (STREET ADDRESS) (CITY & STATE)

Driver's Age _____ Sex _____ Color _____ Driving Exp. ____ Years. Dir.of Travel _____ Speed _____
(OFFICER'S EST)

Driver's Occupation _____ Has driver had High School driver training _____
Place of Employment _____ Address _____
Damage to Car _____ Estimated Amount $ _____
Statement of Driver _____
_____

DAMAGE TO PROPERTY
OTHER THAN VEHICLES _____
(NAME OBJECT AND STATE OF DAMAGE)

NAME AND ADDRESS OF   ESTIMATED
OWNER OF OBJECT STRUCK _____   COST TO REPAIR $ _____

KILLED OR INJURED	OCCUPATION	AGE	MALE FEMALE	PASSENGER PEDESTRIAN	NATURE OF INJURY

1. NAME : _____
ADDRESS: _____
2. NAME : _____
ADDRESS: _____
3. NAME : _____
ADDRESS: _____

Injured were taken to _____ Actual size 8½x11 _____

NAMES AND ADDRESSES OF WITNESSES

1. NAME : _____ ADDRESS: _____ AGE: _____
2. NAME : _____ ADDRESS: _____ AGE: _____
3. NAME : _____ ADDRESS: _____ AGE: _____

STLCO OF P REVISED FORM 9   Form 26   · FOR ADDITIONAL INFORMATION USE FORM 2A

Form 26. Auto.

APPARENT NATURAL DEATH

Call: Subject:
Date:_____   Name _____
Time:_____   Address _____
From whom received: Age_____ Race_____ Sex_____ Occupation_____
_____   Marital Status:___ _____

Found: Time of death:
Where: _____   Witnesses: _____
Date and time: _____   _____
By whom:
                                                Rigor Mortis _____
        (Name and address)   Livor Mortis _____
Other persons
present: _____   Body Temperature _____
_____   Area Temperature _____

Scene: History:
How dressed _____   Past complaints _____
Signs of   When and about what:_____
Violence _____   _____
Visible Wounds
(Yes) (No); If so, describe:_____   Medical treatment _____

Anything suspicious _____   When, for what & by whom:

Medications present _____

Any signs of   Will Doctor sign
Overdose _____   certificate _____

Last seen: PRONOUNCED DEAD
When _____   When _____
By Whom _____   By Whom _____

RELATIVES: _____
Investigation at scene by_____
Cause of Death_____
Disposition _____
REMARKS: _____

_____

APPROVED BY: _____
                                                Coroner's Office
                                                St. Louis County, Missouri

_____
                Coroner
Form 27. Apparent Natural. Actual size 8½ x 14.
(Over for additional information).

MEDICAL EXAMINATION OF A PERSON ALLEGED TO BE DRUNK OR UNDER THE INFLUENCE OF ALCOHOL
(Strike out words not applicable)

Name of person examined _____

Address _____

Occupation _____

Age_____ Sex_____ Race_____

Precise place of examination_____

Examination commenced at_____A.M./P.M. Completed at_____ A.M./P.M., on _____

Whether awake, asleep, or unconscious at time of examination _____

Steps taken to prepare person for examination _____

Conduct of person during such preparation _____

1. Physique of person examined_____   Strong: Weak: Big: Small: Fat: Thin: Normal
2. Pulse (a) _____   Rate_____ Volume_____ Tension_____
3. Pupils (b) _____   Widely, slightly dilated; Normal: Contracted: React normally/sluggishly; Do not react.

    Macewen's sign (c) _____   Present: Absent.
4. Smell of alcohol _____   Strong: Weak: None.
5. Other appearances:
    Conjunctivae _____   Normal: Injected.
    Face _____   Flushed: Normal: Pale.
    Extremities _____   Dry: Moist: Warm: Cold.
    Flow of saliva _____   Profuse: Little: None.
    Vomiting _____   During examination _____
      Signs of past vomiting _____

    Disarrangement of dress _____
6. Gait _____   Staggering: Dragging: Ataxic: Broad Gauge: Normal.

    Romberg's sign _____   Marked: Weak: Absent.
7. Hand movements (picking up objects: finger to finger movement)   Normal: Poor: Bad.
8. Handwriting. Person should sign his/her name in space opposite if able to do so
9. Speech (difficult words and reading few lines of print)   Thick: Slurring: Nasal: Stammering: Normal.
10. Behaviour _____   Noisy: Boasting: Indignant: Insolent: Talkative: Morose: Normal.

11. Orientation (time and place)_____   Good: Moderate: Bad.
12. Memory _____   Clear: Indefinite: Confused.
13. Arithmetical test (depending on education) _____   Good: Moderate: Bad.
14. Temperature _____
15. Describe signs of shock _____   Severe: Mild: None.
16. Signs of injury _____

17. Signs of disease _____

18. Observations (person's own story **only if given voluntarily**). Quantity and type of drink: when and where taken during last 24 hours: time of last meal _____
19. Other remarks _____

NOTE: This form is intended as a guide to medical men when conducting examinations and to prosecutors in leading evidence, and shall not be put in at the trial or preparatory examination. It may be referred to by the medical officer for the purpose of refreshing his memory when giving evidence.

Form 28. Under the Influence of Liquor. Actual size 8½ x 13″.

Time_____

Date_____   No._____

CLOTHING & PERSONAL EFFECTS

Wherever possible, list size, name of manufacturer, Store from which purchased, color, type of material, laundry marks, repair marks and all other pertinent information.

OUTER GARMENTS: _____

_____

_____

_____

_____

_____

_____

UNDER GARMENTS: _____

_____

_____

_____

_____

_____

JEWELRY AND OTHER PERSONAL ITEMS (including watches, rings, keys, pocket knives, etc.):

_____

_____

_____

_____

HANDBAG OR WALLET (Type and contents):_____

_____

_____

_____

_____

_____

_____

Form 29. Clothing and Personal Effects. Actual size 8½ x 14.

F400

ST. LOUIS COUNTY HOSPITAL
Clothing Record

I. Record must be filled out completely in triplicate if clothing is retained in the hospital.
   One record is attached to the patient's record
   One record is attached to the patient's clothing
   One record is placed in E. R. file

II. Record must be filled out completely in duplicate if clothing is released to the proper authorities upon admission of patient into hospital.
   One record is attached to patient's record
   One record is placed in E. R. file

Date ....

Name ....   Hospital No. ....

ARTICLES OF CLOTHING, ETC.	ON ARRIVAL	TAKEN HOME	CLOTHES ROOM	HOSPITAL DIV.	ARTICLES OF CLOTHING, ETC.	ON ARRIVAL	TAKEN HOME	CLOTHES ROOM	HOSPITAL DIV.
Apron					Shirt				
Bathrobe					Skirt				
Belt					Shoes				
Blanket					Shorts				
Blouse					Slip (full)				
Brassiere					Slip (half)				
Cap					Socks				
Coat					Suspenders				
Corset					Sweater				
Diaper					Tie				
Dress					Underpants				
Garters					Undershirt				
Girdle					Union suit				
Gloves					Vest				
Handkerchief					Cane				
Hat					Crutches				
Nose					Dentures (upper)				
Housecoat					Dentures (lower)				
House slippers					Handbag				
Jacket					Partial plate				
Nightgown					Spectacles				
Overcoat					Suitcase				
Pajamas					Truss				
Pants					Prosthesis				
Sanitary belt					Other:				
Scarf									

The undersigned hereby certifies that the above is an accurate and complete list of all clothing brought to St. Louis County Hospital by the patient concerned. All clothing not called for within 90 days following discharge of patient may be disposed of at the discretion of St. Louis County Hospital.

Patient ....   Officer ....

Relative ....   Ambulance Driver ....
(State Relationship)
Signature of one of the above is required

Actual size 8½x11

Clothing listed and checked by (1) ....   } Certification by two hospital }
Hospital Employee   { employees is required   }

(2) ....
Hospital Employee

CLOTHING RELEASED
Date ....

The undersigned hereby certifies that the above listed clothing has been received by the patient concerned or his designated representative and the St. Louis County Hospital is released from any further responsibility.

Patient ....   Officer ....

Relative ....   Ambulance Driver ....
(State Relationship)
Signature of one of the above is required

Witnessed by: (1) ....   Hospital Employee

(2) ....   Hospital Employee

Signature of two hospital employees is required.

Form 30. Clothing Record.

F410

ST. LOUIS COUNTY HOSPITAL
Money and Valuables Record

I. Record must be filled out completely in triplicate if money and/or valuables are retained.
   One record is attached to the patient's record
   One record is attached to money or valuables
   One record is placed in E. R. file

II. Record must be filled out completely in duplicate if money and/or valuables are released to the proper authorities upon admission of patient into hospital.
   One record is attached to patient's record
   One record is placed in E. R. file

Name.. Date..........................

Hospital No..........................

ITEM	NUMBER OF AMOUNT OR ARTICLES	RELEASED TO WARD	RELEASED TO PROPER AUTHORITY	RETAINED IN HOSPITAL	ITEM	AMOUNT OR NUMBER OF ARTICLES	RELEASED TO WARD	RELEASED TO PROPER AUTHORITY	RETAINED IN HOSPITAL
Checks					Ring (set)				
Cash					Ring (band)				
Money Orders					Rosary				
Bank Book					Pin				
Billfold					Pocketbook				
Bracelet					Keys				
Compact					Wristwatch				
Earrings					Other:				
Necklace									

* The hospital does not assume responsibility for any valuables taken to the ward (except a wedding ring and/or one dollar) at the time of patient admission or any other time during his hospital stay. *

The undersigned certifies that the above is an accurate and complete list of all money and valuables brought to St. Louis County Hospital by the patient concerned. If not claimed within 90 days following discharge of patient, these items may be disposed of at the discretion of St. Louis County Hospital.

Patient.. Officer..

Relative..
                (State Relationship)   Ambulance Driver..
                                        Signature of one of the above is required

Checked and listed by (1)..
                        Hospital Employee   { Certification by two hospital }
                                                                             { employees is required }
                    (2)..
                        Hospital Employee

Checked and accepted for deposit by..
                                        Bookkeeper ☐ or Admitting Clerk ☐

Actual size 8½x11

PARTIAL WITHDRAWAL OF MONEY AND VALUABLES

Date..........................

The undersigned certifies that the following articles have been withdrawn:

....

....

Received by.. Witnessed by..

FINAL RELEASE OF MONEY AND VALUABLES

CHECK ONE: Emergency Room ☐   On Discharge from Ward ☐

Date..........................

The undersigned certifies that all of the above listed money and valuables have been received by the patient concerned or his designated representative and that the St. Louis County Hospital is hereby released from all further responsibility.

Patient.. Relative..
                                                        (State Relationship)
                                        Ambulance Driver
Undertaker.. or Officer..
                                        Signature of one of the above is required

Witnessed by: (1) .... (2)..
            Hospital Employee   Hospital Employee
Signature of two hospital employees is required.

Form 31. Money and Valuables Record.

Time_____

Date_____

No._____

REPORT OF A MISSING PERSON AND RECORD OF
IDENTIFICATION

Name _____ Sex_____

_____
(Race)   (Age)   (Height)   (Weight)

Address _____

Occupation _____

When last seen _____

Where _____

Name and address of Relatives (Particularly person reporting subject as missing): _____

_____

_____

_____

General Appearance: _____
                     (Type & Color of Hair) (Type & Color of Eyes

Complexion _____ Type of Beard_____

Shape of:
_____
(Head)   (Nose)   (Eyes)   (Ears)

Physical Characteristics,
such as apparent illnesses _____

    Apparent operations _____

    Scars _____

    Tattoos _____

Teeth: _____
        (Upper)   (Lower)   (Partial)
        (Missing)   (Fillings)   (Defects)

Dentures: _____

List here type of clothing worn by subject when last seen:_____

_____

_____

_____

    This is to certify that on_____, 19____, at_____

(A.M.) (P.M.), I identified_____

in the St. Louis County Morgue, as the above person listed as missing.

                    Name _____

                    Address _____

Witness: _____

Form 32. Report of Missing Person. Actual size 8½ x 14.

Time _____

Date _____

Ambulance _____   No._____

Brought from _____

GENERAL PHYSICAL APPEARANCE

Apparent sex (M) (F) (W) (C)   Approximate Age_____

Measurements of body:

    General Build_____ Waist-line_____

    Height_____ Weight _____

    Shoe Size_____

Type, Cut & Color of Hair_____

Type & Color of Eyes_____

    Glasses, if any_____

Shape of Head_____Nose _____

    Mouth _____Ears _____

Complexion _____Type of Beard_____

Physical characteristics:

    Apparent illness _____

    Apparent operations _____

    Scars _____

    Tattoos _____

Type of Hands _____

Apparent Occupation _____

Teeth _____

    (Missing   (Fillings)   (Defects)

Dentures_____

    (Upper)   (Lower)   (Partial)

X-rays _____

TENTATIVE IDENTIFICATION:

    Name _____

    Address _____

Form 33. General Physical Appearance Report. Actual size 8½ x 14.

FORM TO BE FORWARDED TO PROSECUTING ATTORNEY'S OFFICE

NAME OF DECEASED: _____

DATE, TIME and PLACE OF DEATH:_____

POLICE DEPARTMENT:_____

PATHOLOGIST'S OPINION AS TO CAUSE OF DEATH:_____ _____

_____

_____

WAS INQUEST HELD?_____
(If so, indicate date)

CORONER'S FINDING:_____

_____

_____   _____

_____

___ _____

WITNESSES: _____
(Give Addresses)

_____

_____

___ _____

PHYSICAL EVIDENCE: (Indicate Custody of Same)_____

___ _____

___ _____

___ _____

___ _____   _____

Form 34. Interim Report to Law Enforcement Agency. Actual size 8½ x 13.

_____ COUNTY CORONER'S OFFICE
LABORATORY REPORT
TOXICOLOGICAL EXAMINATION

Case No._____

NAME_____ Autopsy No._____

Date   Date   Date
Procured_____   Received_____   Reported_____

Laboratory No.

	BRAIN	LIVER	KIDNEY	SPLEEN	BLOOD	URINE
VOLATILES						
Acetone						
Aldehydes						
Ethanol						
Methanol						
Phenols						
Cyanides						
Chlorinated Hydrocarbons						
ORGANIC ACIDS						
Barbiturates						
Salicylates						
ORGANIC BASES						
Alkaloid Group Reactions						
HEAVY METALS						
Arsenic						
Lead						
Mercury						

Form 35. Toxicological Examination Report. Actual size 8½ x 11.

ST. LOUIS COUNTY HOSPITAL
Clayton, Mo.

Department of Radiology

X-RAY REPORT

NAME   CASE NO.
ADDRESS   X-RAY NO.
DATE   AGE   SEX

HISTORY

REPORT

Radiologist

Form 36. X-ray Report. Actual size 8½ x 11.

MEDICO-LEGAL REPORT
ST. LOUIS COUNTY CORONER'S OFFICE

Post-mortem Examination   External ( )   Complete ( )

Subject:...

Address:..

Examined at:.. Time.................. Date..................

Age.......... Race....................... Sex....................   DOA   Yes ( )   No ( )

Clinical information known by examiner:...

....

Body length...................... Body weight...................... Decomposition................ ....Rigor......................

Clothing present:...

....

External appearance:...

....Livor Mortis

Marks of Identification...

....

Marks of Violence: Abrasions, contusions, lacerations, fractures, gun shot wounds:...........................

....

....

....

....

....

....

....

....

....

....

....

....

....

....

Present during examination:...

Objects:..

Laboratory Tests:...

....

Conclusions:..

....

....

Date..   Signature...

Form 37.   Medico-Legal Report.

OFFICIAL REPORT OF THE_____COUNTY CORONER

THIS FORM SHOULD ACCOMPANY THE BODY TO COUNTY
CORONER'S OFFICE

FROM_____HOSPITAL

Date_____

STATEMENT AND PARTICULARS IN THE DEATH OF:_____

RESIDENCE_____ Admitted_____ Day of_____
                                      19____, AT_____ A.M._____ P.M.

CONVEYED TO HOSPITAL BY AMBULANCE (____), POLICE (____),

RELATIVE (____), ETC., FROM_____
                              (State whether from public place,
                              jail or residence; give address)

COLOR_____OCCUPATION_____AGE_____Years
                                               _____Months
                                               _____Days

Married, Single, Widowed, Divorced:_____ _____

EXAMINED BY_____ M.D.

Symptoms, subjective and objective, clinical, x-ray and laboratory finding:
(State whether from natural disease, poisoning or injuries. If the latter,
the location, extent, number and character of injuries, whether in shock,
conscious or unconscious)_____

_____

_____

MANNER INJURIES WERE RECEIVED: (Always give such information as will lead to the accurate knowledge of the case and facilitate
judicial inquiry and justice)_____

_____

_____

THERAPY INSTITUTED, INCLUDING OPERATIONS_____

_____

DEATH TOOK PLACE ON THE_____DAY OF___ _____19____
                                                 AT_____
                                                 A.M. P.M.

In your opinion what is the
PROBABLE CAUSE OF DEATH_____ _____

_____

Visiting or resident physician_____
                                                        M.D.

Form 38. Report to Accompany Body to Morgue. Actual size 8½ x 13.

	Box	Bag	Can	Jar	Envelope
Auto Parts		X			
Beer*				X	
Bullets	X				
Billfold					X
Buttons	X				
Bricks		X			
Checks					X
Clothing		X			
Canvas		X			
Capsules	X				
Cartridge cases	X				
Cigarettes	X				
Fibers					X
Firearms					X
Gasoline				X	
Glass	X				
Grass	X				
Hair					X
Headlight Pieces	X				
Handwriting					X
Hat		X			
Ice pick		X			
Ink				X	
Kerosene				X	
Knife		X			
Letters					X
Liquids				X	
Matches (a book of)	X				
Mortar	X				
Paint, chips					X
Paint, liquid				X	
Pills	X				
Plaster	X				
Poison, liquid				X	
Poison, solid	X				
Rags			X		
Safe Insulation	X				
Screen		X			
Screwdriver		X			
Skin tissue	X				
Soil	X				
Thread					X
Tools		X			
Weeds	X				
Whiskey*				X	
Wine*				X	

If there is evidence from the scene (the victim and the subject), place each in a separate container. Seal and label every package.

* Beer, Wine and whiskey in bottles, does not need to be packaged; seal and label only.

Form 39. Evidence Collection Chart. (Actual size 8½ x 11".)

OFFICE OF CORONER
ST. LOUIS COUNTY, MISSOURI

Date_____19____

Received from_____

the following Personal Property regarding the death of _____

_____

Cash_____Valuables_____

_____

_____

_____

_____

_____
(Relationship to Deceased)

Address:_____

_____(Witness)

Address_____

Form 40. Receipt for Possessions and Evidence.

ST. LOUIS COUNTY CORONER

Time_____   RE:_____

Date_____   Name_____

In person ☐   Call from ☐   Call to ☐   Information ☐   Inquiry ☐

NOTES:

Actual size 5½x8¼

Form 41. Record of Phone Calls and Inquiries.

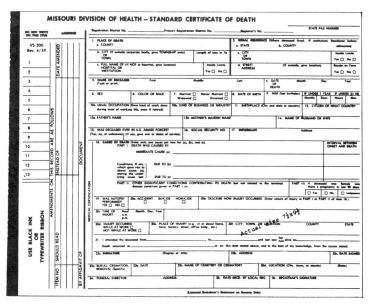

Form 42. Standard Death Certificate.

THE DIVISION OF HEALTH OF MISSOURI

STANDARD CERTIFICATE OF FETAL DEATH

STATE FILE NUMBER

Dept. Health,
Educ., & Welfare
U. S. Public
Health Service

V. S. 375
Rev. 9-35

Registration District No................. Primary Registration District No................. Registrar's No........ ....

A child born dead after 20 weeks gestation will be reported on this form.

Fetuses unclaimed or used for medical purposes shall be reported to the State Anatomical Board, Columbia, Missouri, in addition to filing this report with the local registrar.

Person responsible for caring for remains must file this report within 3 days after delivery and receive local registrar's permit for disposition.

WRITE PLAINLY - UNFADING BLACK INK - MAKE A PERMANENT RECORD

1 PLACE OF DELIVERY				2. USUAL RESIDENCE OF MOTHER (Where does mother live?)			
a. COUNTY				a. STATE		b. COUNTY	
b. CITY (If outside corporate limits, give TOWNSHIP only) OR TOWN		Inside Limits Yes ☐ No ☐		c. CITY OR TOWN			Inside Limits Yes ☐ No ☐
c. FULL NAME OF (If NOT in hospital or institution, give street address or location) HOSPITAL OR INSTITUTION				d. STREET ADDRESS	(If outside, give location)		Reside on Form Yes ☐ No ☐

3 NAME OF FETUS (if given)		4. SEX OF FETUS MALE ☐ FEMALE ☐ UNDETERMINED ☐

5a. THIS DELIVERY SINGLE ☐ TWIN ☐ TRIPLET ☐	5b. IF TWIN OR TRIPLET WAS THIS FETUS DELIVERED 1ST ☐ 2ND ☐ 3RD ☐	6. DATE OF DELIVERY (Month) (Day) (Year)

FATHER	7 NAME a. (First) b. (Middle) c. (Last)		8 COLOR OR RACE
	9 AGE (At time of delivery) YEARS	10 BIRTHPLACE (State or foreign country)	11a. USUAL OCCUPATION 11b. KIND OF BUSINESS OR INDUSTRY
MOTHER	12 MAIDEN NAME a. (First) b. (Middle) c. (Last)		13 COLOR OR RACE
	14 AGE (At time of delivery) YEARS	15 BIRTHPLACE (State or foreign country)	16. PREVIOUS DELIVERIES TO MOTHER (Do NOT include this fetus)

16. PREVIOUS DELIVERIES TO MOTHER (Do NOT include this fetus)
a. How many children are now living?
b. How many children were born alive but are now dead?
c. How many PREVIOUS fetal deaths (fetuses born dead at ANY time after conception)?

17 INFORMANT	

18a. LENGTH OF PREGNANCY COMPLETED .... WEEKS	18b. WEIGHT OF FETUS ...... LB ...... OZ	19 LEGITIMATE YES ☐ NO ☐	20 WHEN DID FETUS DIE BEFORE LABOR ☐ DURING LABOR OR DELIVERY ☐ UNKNOWN ☐	21 AUTOPSY YES ☐ NO ☐

22. CAUSE OF FETAL DEATH	I DIRECT AND ANTECEDENT CAUSES	(Enter only one cause per line)	
	DIRECT CAUSE *State fetal or maternal condition directly causing fetal death (do not use such terms as stillbirth or prematurity).*	(a)	
	ANTECEDENT CAUSES. *State fetal and/or maternal conditions, if any, GIVING RISE TO THE ABOVE CAUSE (a) stating THE UNDERLYING CAUSE LAST.*	Due to (b)	
		Due to (c)	

Actual size 8½ x 7½

II OTHER SIGNIFICANT CONDITIONS of fetus or mother which may have CONTRIBUTED to fetal death, but, in so far as is known, were not related to direct cause of fetal death		23. SYPHILIS TEST Yes ☐ No ☐

I hereby certify that this delivery occurred on the date stated above and the fetus was born dead.	24a. ATTENDANT'S SIGNATURE	(Specify if M. D., D. O., midwife, or other)	24b. DATE SIGNED
	24c. ATTENDANT'S ADDRESS	If not attended by physician	25. SIGNATURE OF AUTHORIZED OFFICIAL TITLE

26a. BURIAL, CREMATION, REMOVAL (Specify)	26b. DATE	26c. NAME OF CEMETERY OR CREMATORY	26d. LOCATION (City, town, or county) (State)

27. PERSON IN CHARGE OF DISPOSITION ADDRESS	DATE REC'D BY LOCAL. REG.	REGISTRAR'S SIGNATURE

(Licensed Embalmer's Statement on Reverse Side)

Form 43. Fetal Death Certificate.

AUTOPSY CONSENT

Date_____

I hereby authorize the Coroner of_____
County, State of Missouri (or his Deputy), to make a postmortem examination or autopsy in the case of

_____
(Name)   (Address in Full)

who is my_____
(Relationship of Deceased to One Granting Permit)

(Signed)_____

_____
(Address in Full)

Witness:

_____

_____
(Address in Full)

Form 44. Autopsy Consent Form.

GROUP	TYPICAL COMMON POISON	FATAL DOSE

ACIDS
   ACETIC
   SULFURIC
   NITRIC
   . . . .
 ALKALIS
   AMMONIA
   POTASSIUM
   (HYDROXIDE
   . . . .
   ALKALINE
   (CARBONATES
	(1) **MURIATIC**
	
	 (2) **LYE**
		Unavailable . . . as no Official doses exist, save in case of Conc. U.S.P. acids, which have maximum of $_m$10

ARSENIC
   PARIS GREEN
 	
   FLY PAPERS
     some
   RAT POISONS
	(3) **SODIUM ARSENATE**	Not available
		
		 Maximum Medicinal dose . . . 1/20th gr.

ALKALOIDS
   RAT POISONS
 	
   COUGH MIX-
     TURES
	(4) **STRYCHNINE**
	
	 (5) **MORPHINE**
	     CODEINE
		Strychnine . . . FATAL DOSE between ½ and 1 gr.
		
		 Morphine about 30 mg.

CAMPHOR
   LINIMENTS
 	
   PAREGORIC
	OPIUM &
	 (6) **CAMPHOR**
		Mortality low—no fatal dose available
		
		 As Morphine (2½ fl. ozs.)

GASES
   ACETYLENE
   AUTO EXHAUST
 	
   BLEACH
   CLOROX
 	
   PUREX
	(7) **CARBON MONOXIDE**
	
	 (8) **CHLORINE**	

Form 45. Poison Chart.

SYMPTOMS OF POISONING
(Characteristic Symptoms in Bold)

Recognized by presence of burns about mouth, corrosion of membranes (mucous) of mouth, throat & oesophagus, "Coffee-Ground" vomit. Later, intense swelling of throat, mouth, oesophagus. Clammy skin, rapid, feeble pulse.

Often perforation & stricture, Cardiac failure.

Litmus paper to vomitus, or excreta determines whether Acid, or Alkali.

(N.B. Blue Litmus changes to Red with Acid. Red Litmus to Blue with Alkali.)

Vomiting, profuse diarrhoea, "RICE WATER" stools & bloody discharges. "GARLICKY" odour of breath and stools.

Cyanosis, circulatory collapse, convulsions, coma.

Muscular twitching & rigidity, muscles jerk on touch. Tetanic convulsions every 3-30 min. Eyeballs rolled up. "RISUS SARDONICUS." Paralysis. Death from asphyxia. Body arched backwards.

"Pin point Pupils," jaw falls. "Cheyne Stokes" breathing. Retention of urine, cyanosis, convulsions—especially in children. Pupils now dilate, then death.

CAMPHOR: Characteristic odour of breath with both Liniments & Paregoric & Urine. Vomiting, circulatory collapse.

PAREGORIC. As symptoms for Camphor & Opium (under Alkaloids, above.)

CARBON MONOXIDE. Skin dusky, lips often blue. Marked muscular rigidity (particularly jaw). Victim never entirely blue, even when asphyxiation complete. Apnoea,—Coma.

CHLORINE. Corrosion of mouth. Distressing spasmodic cough, possible perforation, Circulatory Collapse.

GROUP	TYPICAL COMMON POISON	FATAL DOSE
OXALATES STRAW HAT CLEANER BRASS POLISH	(9) **OXALIS ACID**	Unavailable
PHENOLS CARBOLIC ACID CRESOL DISINFECTANTS LYSOL	(10) **CRESOL**	
PHOSPHORUS MATCHES SOME RAT POISONS	(11) **RAT POISON**	NOT AVAILABLE in terms of matches
SALICYLATES ASPIRIN SODIUM SALICYLATE METHYL SALICYLATE	(12) **ASPIRIN**	Doses of from 30-90 five gr. Aspirin Tabs usually fatal

HYPNOTICS

BARBITURATES PHENOBARBITAL AMYTAL SODIUM AMYTAL BARBITONE BUINAL NEMBUTAL (or Pentobarbital)	(13) **NEMBUTAL**	Amytal 30-45 gr. Barbitone (75-200 gr.) Nembutal (over 30 gr.) Phenobarbital (90-150 gr.)

NOTE: Many of these "fatal doses" are inconclusive. Generally speaking, when poison is of a corrosive nature . . . e.g., Oxalic Acid, or even Phosphorus poisons . . . "dosage is inapplicable."
In the case of Carbolic Acid, while it has an extremely small medicinal dose, well, diluted . . . in large undiluted amounts, it is a corrosive.

Form 45. Poison Chart.

SYMPTOMS OF POISONING
(Characteristic Symptoms in Bold)

Gastro-intestinal irritation. Vomiting, usually bloody. Twitching of facial muscles. Cold cyanotic skin. Dilated pupils. Convulsions—Coma.

Characteristic odour on breath. Local necrosis of lips & mouth,—first white, then brown. Salivation. Vomiting rare. Vertigo. **Urine black on standing.** Face & skin livid & clammy. Fall in blood pressure & body temperature. Death from respiratory failure, or possibly oedema of glottis & lungs.

Garlicky breath odour, vomitus bloody or coffee colored & luminous in dark, with **garlicky** odour. Bloody diarrhoea. If victim survives, quiescent period of 1-3 days, followed by vomiting, diarrhoea, pruritis, enlarged liver, ecchymosis, vertigo, thready pulse. Collapse, coma, haematuria, convulsions.

Vomiting, epigastric pain. With Methyl Salicyl. Odour of Wintergreen. Delirium, hallucinations. Pallor, skin eruptions. Kussamul's reaction (or Airhunger) due to acidosis. Urine gives "salicylate reaction" with **Ferris Chloride (port-wine color)** NOT removed by boiling.

Mental confusion, etaxia (twitching of muscles). History of falls, accidents & slurring of speech. Delirium, at first quiet-deepening into come. Respiration at first quiet & slow, then shallow & slow, then noisy. Cyanosis. Absence of corneal & other reflexes. Occasional hippus. Anuria & circulatory collapse. Blood pressure low. Death usually after several days unconsciousness, from pulmonary oedema,—the pneumonia accompanied by fever & other classic signs.

NOTE: Symptoms of the subject before his death should be determined by the Police Officer in his questioning and investigation, firstly, to indicate if any of the above poisons was taken and, secondly, to give the pathologist and medical technologist an idea for which poison to test.

FETUS

CM. LENGTH RELATED TO AGE:			GM WEIGHT RELATED TO AGE:
Crown-Rump	*Crown-Heel*	*Lunar Month*	
− 2.3	− 3.0	Second	1.1 − 3.5
5.1 − 7.4	7.0 − 9.8	Third	14.0 − 14.3
10.7 − 11.6	15.5 − 18.0	Fourth	86.8 − 108.0
15.5 − 16.4	22.7 − 25.0	Fifth	260.0 − 316.0
19.7 − 20.8	29.2 − 31.5	Sixth	551.0 − 630.0
23.6 − 24.7	35.0 − 37.1	Seventh	971.0 − 1,045.0
27.1 − 28.3	40.4 − 42.5	Eighth	1,519.0 − 1,680.0
30.5 − 32.1	45.4 − 47.0	Ninth	2,196.0 − 2,378.0
33.6 − 36.2	50.0 − 50.2	Tenth	2,998.0 − 3,405.0

Form 46. Fetus (Determination of Age).

I. Purpose
  A. To check questionable stains where collection difficult
     AND
  B. To disprove presumption that stain is blood.
  C. Does not definitely establish that stain is blood

II. Steps
  A. Fill test tube or small bottle with inch of distilled water.
  B. Add one-half gram of benzidine dihydrochloride.
  C. Shake well until dissolved.
  D. Add one cubic centimeter of 3% peroxide.
  E. Shake again.
  F. Collect part of stain on piece of filter paper.
  G. Place few drops of solution on stain.
  H. If stain is blood, bluish-green color appears.

III. Confirmation
  A. Collect additional stain as evidence
     AND
  B. Submit to laboratory for confirmation that
     1. It is blood;
     2. It is human (?) blood;
     3. Blood groups.

Note: Test will definitely establish that stain is blood, but will not definitely establish that it is blood.

Form 47.   Benzedine Test for Blood.

FIREARMS, RESIDUE, IDENTIFICATION
HARRISON METHOD

Step	Instructions	Results
1.	Take a 2″ square of cloth and moisten with 0.1 molar hydrochloric acid solution	
2.	Swab the specific area of the hand	
3.	Dry the cloth thoroughly	
4.	Apply 1 to 2 drops of 10% alcoholic solution of triphenylmethylarsonium iodide	Orange color develops in 30 seconds; to full color in 2 minutes, thus confirming the presence of antimony
5.	Dry the cloth thoroughly. Add 1 to 2 drops of 5% solution sodium rhodizonate to orange color	Red color develops, confirming presence of barium and lead
6.	Dry cloth thoroughly. Add 1 to 2 drops of 1:20 hydrochloric acid to sheet of cloth containing the red color	Blue color develops inside the ring, confirming the presence of lead. If a red color remains inside the blue area, it confirms the presence of barium.

Form 48. Firearms Residue Identification.

PARAFFIN METHOD

1. Melt paraffin.

2. Spread or pour over finger, hand or rest of individual being examined, until a coating of paraffin ⅛″ thick is obtained.

3. When parafin is cool, cast is pulled gently from the hand.

4. Apply reagent made by adding (with constant stirring) 10 ml of concentrated sulphuric acid to 2 ml of distilled water. To this solution 0.05 gms of diphenylamine should be added and stirred until completely dissolved.

5. Positive re-action is indicated by appearance of dark blue specks (interfering substances composed of nitrates such as tranquilizers, urine, certain foods, bleaching agents, etcetera, may also give a positive result).

Form 49. Paraffin Residue Identification.

REFERENCES

Mack, William, and Kiser, Donald: *Corpus Juris Secundum.* American Law Book Company, Brooklyn, New York, Copyright 1936.

Dorland, W. A. Newman: *The American Illustrated Medical Dictionary.* W. B. Saunders Co., Philadelphia and London, 1951.

Gray, Roscoe N.: *Attorneys' Textbook of Medicine—Third Edition.* Mathews, Berle & Co., Albany and New York, 1961.

Polson, C. J.: Brittain, R. P., and Marshall, T. K.: *The Disposal of the Dead.* Philosophical Library, Inc., New York, 1953.

Gordon, I.; Turner, R., and Price, T. W.: *Medical Jurisprudence—Third Edition.* E. & S. Livingstone, Ltd., Edinburgh and London, 1953.

Snyder, LeMoyne: *Homicide Investigation.* Charles C Thomas, Publisher, Springfield, Ill., 1959.

Camps, F. E., and Purchas, W. B.: *Practical Forensic Medicine.* The MacMillan Co., New York, 1957.

Southwestern Law Enforcement Institute on Homicide Investigation Techniques. Charles C Thomas, Publisher, Springfield, Ill., 1961.

Soderman, Harry, and O'Connell, John J.: *Modern Criminal Investigation.* Funk & Wagnalls Co., New York and London, 1940.

Judge and Prosecutor in Traffic Court, Northwestern Institute. American Bar Association and Northwestern University, 1951.

Merkeley, Donald Carl: *The Investigation of Death.* Charles C Thomas, Publisher, Springfield, Ill., 1957.

Proceedings of Seminars of National Association of Coroners— 1954, 1955, 1956, 1957, 1958, 1959 and 1960.

357

O'Hara, Charles E.: *Fundamentals of Criminal Investigation.* Charles C Thomas, Publisher, Springfield, Illinois, 1956.

Gonzales, T.; Vance, M.; Helpern, M., and Umberger, C.: *Legal Medicine, Pathology and Toxicology.* Appleton Century Croft Co., New York, 1954.

Mant, A. Keith: *Forensic Medicine.* The Year Book Publishers, Inc., Chicago, Ill., 1960.

Gerber, Sam: *The Scope and Problems of the Coroner*—Cleveland Ohio, 1950.

Tuttle, Harris: *Criminal Photography.* Rochester, New York.

Department of Public Health of Illinois: *Manual for Coroners,* 1959.

Department of Public Health of Illinois: *Manual for Coroners' Physicians,* 1959.

Department of Public Health of Illinois: *Manual for Pathologists,* 1960.

Garnholz, Edward W. (Prosecuting Attorney): *Handbook on Crime.* St. Louis County, Missouri, 1958.

Svensson, Arne, and Wendell, Otto: *Crime Detection.* Elsevier Publishing Co., Amsterdam, Houston, London and New York, 1955.

State of Missouri Civil Defense Agency: *Civil Defense Police Services.* Jefferson City, Missouri, 1952.

INDEX